WALL PILATES

WORKOUT FOR WOMENS

Tone and Strengthen your Muscles and
Enhance Mental Wellbeing

Woman Tailored Workout. Results in 4 weeks with Few minutes per Day
Anytime, Anywhere

By Jada Larkfield

TABLE OF CONTENTS

Introduction: unlocking the power of Wall Pilates

At the heart of Wall Pilates lies a transformative journey that goes beyond mere physical exercise; it's a holistic approach to wellness that taps into the power of the mind-body connection. In this in-depth exploration, we unravel the layers of Wall Pilates, delving into its core principles, unique methodology, and the profound impact it can have on your overall well-being.

Wall Pilates is built upon a foundation of core principles that serve as the guiding light for practitioners. These principles, including breath control, core engagement, and mindful movement, lay the groundwork for a practice that goes beyond superficial fitness goals. The integration of these principles fosters a deep sense of awareness, connecting the mind and body in a symbiotic dance.

Unlike conventional workouts that may prioritize external results, Wall Pilates places emphasis on internal transformation. It's not just about the physical postures but about cultivating a mindful presence throughout each movement. This mind-body harmony distinguishes Wall Pilates as a practice that nurtures both the physical and mental aspects of well-being.

The Supportive Wall: A Pillar of Strength for Beginners

Central to the uniqueness of Wall Pilates is the integration of a supportive wall. For beginners, the wall becomes a pillar of strength, offering stability and assistance as they navigate through foundational exercises. This accessibility makes Wall Pilates an inviting entry point for individuals of all fitness levels, even those who may feel intimidated by more advanced workouts.

The wall serves as a constant companion, instilling confidence in practitioners as they build strength and flexibility. It acts as a supportive partner, allowing individuals to focus on form and precision without the fear of instability. This symbiotic relationship with the wall fosters a sense of trust, creating a safe space for exploration and growth.

Precision in Every Move: Mastering the Basics

While Wall Pilates welcomes beginners with open arms, it also challenges seasoned practitioners by emphasizing precision in every move. Mastery of the basics becomes a continuous journey, with the wall providing both resistance and refinement. The controlled and deliberate nature of Wall Pilates movements elevates it from a simple workout to an artful practice.

In the pursuit of mastering the basics, practitioners not only sculpt and strengthen their bodies but also fine-tune their awareness. The wall becomes a responsive partner, offering feedback and resistance that encourages practitioners to delve deeper into their practice. This commitment to precision sets Wall Pilates apart as a dynamic and evolving discipline.

Beyond the physical postures and principles, Wall Pilates holds transformative powers that extend into various facets of life. It becomes a metaphorical canvas where individuals paint strokes of resilience, self-discovery, and empowerment. The wall, once a source of support, transforms into a mirror reflecting the strength that resides within.

The transformative journey in Wall Pilates is not confined to the studio; it permeates daily life. Practitioners discover newfound confidence, improved posture, and a heightened sense of body awareness that transcends the mat. This decoding of Wall Pilates unravels its potential to be a lifelong companion in the pursuit of holistic well-being.

In essence, the overview of Wall Pilates is an invitation to embark on a journey that transcends the conventional boundaries of fitness. It's a pathway to self-discovery, where the supportive wall becomes a silent ally in the exploration of physical and mental strength. As we navigate the chapters ahead, each layer of Wall Pilates unfolds, revealing a practice that not only transforms bodies but empowers lives.

Wall Pilates vs. Yoga and Traditional Pilates: Understanding the Differences

Embarking on a wellness journey often involves navigating through a myriad of fitness modalities, each with its unique philosophy and methodology. In the realm of mind-body exercises, Wall Pilates stands out as a transformative practice that shares common ground with both Yoga and Traditional Pilates while carving its distinct path. Let's delve into the distinctive dimensions of Wall Pilates, Yoga, and Traditional Pilates to unravel the nuances that shape these practices.

Wall Pilates: A Fusion of Stability and Support

Wall Pilates, at its core, is a contemporary adaptation of traditional Pilates that integrates the support of a wall. While grounded in the foundational principles of Pilates, such as core engagement, breath control, and mindful movement, Wall Pilates introduces a dynamic element by utilizing the wall as a stabilizing force. The wall serves as a dependable partner, offering support and resistance, thereby enhancing the precision and effectiveness of movements.

In Wall Pilates, the wall acts as a multifunctional prop, providing stability for beginners and challenging resistance for advanced practitioners. This fusion of stability and support sets Wall Pilates apart, making it accessible to a broad audience, including those who may find traditional Pilates challenging.

Yoga: The Harmony of Mind, Body, and Spirit

Yoga, an ancient practice with roots in Indian philosophy, transcends the realms of physical exercise. It is a holistic approach that seeks to harmonize the mind, body, and spirit. Yoga encompasses various styles, each emphasizing different aspects, such as Hatha for physical postures, Vinyasa for flow, and Kundalini for spiritual awakening.

Unlike Pilates, Yoga often incorporates meditation, breathwork (pranayama), and spiritual elements. While both Yoga and Wall Pilates promote mind-body connection, Yoga places a stronger emphasis on holistic well-being and spiritual growth. The fluidity of Yoga movements contrasts with the precise and controlled nature of Wall Pilates exercises.

Traditional Pilates: Precision and Control

Traditional Pilates, developed by Joseph Pilates in the early 20th century, focuses on strengthening the core, improving flexibility, and promoting overall body awareness. Pilates exercises are characterized by precision, control, and flowing movements. The emphasis on the powerhouse—core muscles—sets Traditional Pilates apart as a sculpting and toning practice.

Unlike Wall Pilates, which integrates the support of a wall, Traditional Pilates primarily utilizes specialized equipment such as the reformer, Cadillac, and barrel. This equipment provides variable resistance and assistance, allowing practitioners to tailor the intensity of exercises. Traditional Pilates is renowned for its ability to enhance posture, flexibility, and muscle tone.

Bridging the Gap: The Unique Essence of Wall Pilates

While Wall Pilates shares common ground with Yoga and Traditional Pilates, its unique essence lies in the fusion of stability, support, and adaptability. The wall becomes a constant companion, offering a sense of security for beginners while providing resistance for those seeking a more challenging workout. The adaptability of Wall Pilates makes it suitable for individuals of all fitness levels, ages, and body types.

In contrast to Yoga's spiritual depth and Traditional Pilates' equipment-based precision, Wall Pilates distinguishes itself through simplicity and accessibility. The wall becomes a versatile prop that facilitates exercises without the need for complex equipment, making it an ideal practice for those seeking a balanced fusion of strength, flexibility, and mindful movement.

In conclusion, while Wall Pilates draws inspiration from the foundational principles of Traditional Pilates and shares a mind-body connection with Yoga, it stands as a unique and adaptable practice. The incorporation of the wall as a supportive element transforms the Pilates experience, making it inclusive, effective, and accessible to a diverse audience on their wellness journey. Whether you are drawn to the precision of Traditional Pilates, the holistic approach of Yoga, or seeking a versatile and supportive practice, Wall Pilates invites you to explore a transformative path that resonates with your individual needs and goals.

Chapter 1: Foundation of Wall Pilates

Welcome to the foundational realm of Wall Pilates, where the essence of your transformative journey begins. In this chapter, we delve into the core principles that serve as the bedrock of Wall Pilates, crafting the framework for a practice that transcends the ordinary.

Unlocking the Core Principles: A Deeper Dive

The core principles of Wall Pilates are not mere guidelines; they're the secret language your body speaks during each session. Precision, the art of exactness in movement, ensures that every action serves a purpose. Control, the mastery over your body, transforms exercises into a journey of self-discovery. Centering is the gravitational force that grounds your energy, fostering stability and balance.

Concentration becomes your superpower, allowing you to channel your focus entirely into the present moment. Breath is the life force that sustains you throughout the practice, and flow, the seamless transition between movements, creates a dance that feels as effortless as it is transformative. As you delve into each principle, you unlock the alchemy that makes Wall Pilates a profound experience.

Crafting Your Pilates Sanctuary: Beyond the Physical Space

Your Pilates space isn't just a physical location; it's a state of mind. Learn to infuse your practice area with elements that inspire and uplift. Whether it's soft lighting, soothing music, or personal mementos, your Pilates sanctuary becomes a reflection of your inner journey. It's a space where the boundaries between the external and internal blur, allowing you to tap into a profound sense of self.

Mindful Movement Unveiled: The Poetry of Pilates

Explore the poetry in Pilates through mindful movement. This goes beyond the technical execution of exercises. It's an invitation to feel each stretch, engage with each muscle, and savor the fluidity of transitions. In this section, discover the magic that happens when movement becomes a conscious, intentional act. Wall Pilates is not just about doing; it's about being present in every nuance of your physical exploration.

By cultivating a dance-like rhythm between breath and body, you elevate your practice beyond the physical, entering a realm where each movement becomes a meditation, and every breath propels you deeper into the flow.

Guided Meditation: A Journey Within

The mind-body connection is a treasure waiting to be unearthed. Through a guided meditation, embark on a journey within. This isn't about emptying the mind; it's about filling it with awareness. Dive into the stillness, connect with your breath, and explore the profound dialogue between your mental landscape and physical sensations. This meditation isn't a separate entity; it's a seamless extension of your Pilates practice, enriching every aspect of your being.

As you immerse yourself in the foundational aspects of Wall Pilates, you're not just learning exercises; you're initiating a dialogue with your body, mind, and space. Each principle, every mindful movement, and the guided meditation are threads in the tapestry of your Pilates journey, weaving together a narrative of self-discovery, balance, and transformative growth.

Chapter 2: Debunking Myths - The Truth About Wall Pilates

Myth 1: Pilates is Only for the Flexible

In unraveling this myth, we discover that flexibility is not a prerequisite but a reward of consistent Pilates practice. Wall Pilates accommodates all levels, gradually enhancing flexibility without demanding it from the start.

Myth 2: No Equipment Means No Results

Contrary to this notion, Wall Pilates harnesses the support of the wall, making it a powerful tool. The absence of complex equipment doesn't diminish its effectiveness; rather, it simplifies your journey, focusing on precise movements and body control.

Myth 3: Wall Pilates is not Intense Enough for a Good Workout

Prepare to challenge this belief as Wall Pilates proves that intensity isn't synonymous with high impact. Through controlled movements and strategic engagement, it delivers a holistic workout that builds strength, endurance, and flexibility.

Myth 4: Pilates Won't Build Muscle or Aid Weight Loss

This myth crumbles under the weight of evidence that Pilates, including the wall variant, significantly contributes to muscle toning and weight management. The emphasis on controlled resistance and targeted muscle engagement fuels both aspects of physical transformation.

Myth 5: Pilates is Only for Rehabilitation

While Pilates indeed aids in rehabilitation, its scope extends far beyond. It serves as a proactive means to prevent injuries, enhance performance, and sculpt a resilient body capable of meeting life's demands.

Myth 6: Pilates Won't Benefit Cardiovascular Health

Contrary to popular belief, Wall Pilates incorporates dynamic movements that elevate heart rate and promote cardiovascular health. While it may not mirror traditional cardio exercises, its comprehensive benefits extend to heart health and overall well-being.

Myth 7: Wall Pilates Only Targets the Core

Beyond the core, Wall Pilates engages multiple muscle groups. From legs to arms, it sculpts the entire body, fostering balanced strength and endurance. The core is pivotal, but it's just the starting point of a holistic transformation.

Myth 8: Pilates is a Passing Fitness Trend

With decades of endurance, Pilates, including Wall Pilates, stands as a timeless practice rooted in its transformative efficacy. It has proven to be not a trend, but a sustainable lifestyle choice embraced by fitness enthusiasts worldwide.

Myth 9: Wall Pilates is Only for Women

Wall Pilates is inclusive, offering benefits to everyone, regardless of gender. Dispelling the notion that it's exclusively for women, it welcomes individuals seeking a mindful, effective, and adaptable workout routine.

Myth 10: You Need to Be Young to Practice Wall Pilates

Age is not a barrier; it's an ally in Wall Pilates. Tailored to accommodate all age groups, this myth collapses as Wall Pilates becomes a fountain of youth, promoting strength, flexibility, and well-being at any stage of life.

By dismantling these myths, we pave the way for a more inclusive understanding of Wall Pilates, revealing its universal accessibility and transformative potential for individuals of all backgrounds and fitness levels.

Chapter 3: Motivation for Your Pilates Journey

In this chapter, the narratives of real women seamlessly intertwine with the goals, challenges, and aspirations of our female avatars. Their stories echo the sentiments of countless women seeking solace, strength, and transformation through Wall Pilates.

Female Avatars Speak: Real Stories of Transformation

Meet Emma Thompson, a 33-year-old marketing executive and busy mother of two. Emma's goal was clear—to regain her pre-pregnancy fitness and find a sustainable workout routine amidst her bustling life. With Wall Pilates, she not only achieved physical transformation but discovered newfound energy to keep up with her active family. Emma's journey resonates with women like our avatar, highlighting the tangible results achievable through dedication and the right fitness approach.

Overcoming Skepticism: Finding Motivation Within

Sarah Carter, a 28-year-old artist, initially harbored skepticism about the efficacy of Wall Pilates. Juggling her artistic pursuits and part-time job, Sarah doubted if a seemingly simple practice could yield meaningful results. However, as she embraced the discipline and witnessed her body's transformation, Sarah's skepticism turned into unwavering belief. Her story mirrors the initial reservations many women harbor and dismantles the myth that effective fitness requires elaborate equipment or intense workouts.

Pilates and Emotional Well-being: Building a Positive Body Connection

Diana Rodriguez, a 40-year-old IT professional, found herself grappling with emotional well-being and body image concerns. Pilates wasn't just about physical exercise for Diana; it became a sanctuary where she cultivated a positive connection with her body. Her journey sheds light on the emotional impact of Wall Pilates, providing a holistic approach to well-being that resonates with those facing similar challenges.

Staying Committed: Practical Tips for Daily Practice

Stella Martin, a 45-year-old entrepreneur and avid traveler, encountered the perennial challenge of staying committed to a fitness routine amid a dynamic lifestyle. Stella's story outlines practical tips she discovered on her Pilates journey—carving out dedicated time, incorporating Pilates into her travel routine, and celebrating the small wins. Her insights are a beacon for women seeking realistic ways to integrate Pilates into their daily lives.

These authentic stories breathe life into the very essence of our female avatars' goals, challenges, and frustrations. Emma, Sarah, Diana, and Stella showcase that Wall Pilates is not just an exercise routine but a catalyst for transformative change—both physical and emotional. Their narratives offer a roadmap for women looking to embark on a Pilates journey that aligns with their unique aspirations and life circumstances.

Chapter 4: Foundation Fitness Assessment - Tailoring Wall Pilates to YOU

"Unlock Your Potential: Easy and Beginner-Friendly Tests to Personalize Your Wall Pilates Experience"
This chapter serves as your gateway to a personalized Wall Pilates journey.

We believe in meeting you where you are, and that's why we've included a series of easy and beginner-friendly fitness tests. These tests will help you understand your current physical fitness level, allowing you to tailor your Wall Pilates practice for optimal results. From mobility to strength, discover the key aspects of your fitness and embark on a journey that's uniquely yours. Let's lay the groundwork for a transformative experience.

Let's expand on each subsection with instructions, objectives, and objective values for the 10 beginner-friendly fitness tests:

1 - Flexibility Test - Toe Touch

Instructions:
- Stand with feet hip-width apart.
- Slowly bend forward at the waist and try to touch your toes.
- Note how far you can reach comfortably.

Objective:
Assess the flexibility of the hamstrings and lower back.
Objective Values:
- Excellent: Palms touch the floor.
- Good: Fingertips reach below knees.
- Average: Fingertips reach mid-shin.
- Below Average: Fingertips above mid-shin.

2 - Core Strength Test - Plank

Instructions:
- Assume a push-up position with arms straight.
- Keep your body in a straight line from head to heels.
- Hold the plank position for 30 seconds to a minute.

Objective:
Evaluate core strength and endurance.
Objective Values:
- Excellent: Maintain for 1 minute.
- Good: Hold for 45 seconds.
- Average: Hold for 30 seconds.
- Below Average: Hold for less than 30 seconds.

3 - Balance Test - Single Leg Stand

Instructions:
- Stand on one leg and lift the other leg a few inches off the ground.

- Try to maintain balance for 30 seconds.
- Repeat on the other leg.
- Do this with eye open and then with eye closed.

Objective:
Test overall balance and stability.
Objective Values:
- Excellent: Maintain balance for 30 seconds on both legs.
- Good: Stable for 20-30 seconds on each leg.
- Average: Stable for 10-20 seconds on each leg.
- Below Average: Less than 10 seconds on each leg.

4 - Upper Body Strength Test - Wall Push-Up

Instructions:
- Stand facing a wall and place your hands on the wall at shoulder height.
- Perform push-ups against the wall, ensuring a straight line from head to heels.

Objective:
Assess upper body strength.
Objective Values:
- Excellent: Perform 20 or more push-ups.
- Good: Perform 10-20 push-ups.
- Average: Perform 5-10 push-ups.
- Below Average: Perform less than 5 push-ups.

5 - Lower Body Strength Test - Wall Sit

Instructions:
- Stand with your back against a wall and lower your body into a seated position.
- Aim for a 90-degree angle at the knees and hold the position for 30 seconds.

Objective:
Evaluate lower body strength and endurance.
Objective Values:
- Excellent: Hold for 1 minute.
- Good: Hold for 45 seconds.
- Average: Hold for 30 seconds.
- Below Average: Hold for less than 30 seconds.

6 - Mobility Test - Neck Rotation

Instructions:
- Slowly turn your head to the left and then to the right.
- Note any stiffness or discomfort.

Objective:
Assess neck mobility.

Objective Values:
- Excellent: Full range of motion with no discomfort.
- Good: Full range of motion with mild discomfort.
- Average: Limited range of motion with moderate discomfort.
- Below Average: Limited range of motion with significant discomfort.

7 - Cardiovascular Test - March in Place

Instructions:
- March in place for 2 minutes, lifting your knees as high as comfortable.
- Assess your ability to sustain the activity without excessive fatigue.

Objective:
Evaluate cardiovascular endurance.
Objective Values:
- Excellent: Complete 2 minutes without fatigue.
- Good: Complete 1.5-2 minutes with mild fatigue.
- Average: Complete 1-1.5 minutes with moderate fatigue.
- Below Average: Less than 1 minute.

8 - Breathing Test - Diaphragmatic Breathing

Instructions:
- Lie on your back and place one hand on your chest and the other on your abdomen.
- Inhale deeply, allowing your abdomen to rise more than your chest.

Objective:
Focus on diaphragmatic breathing.
Objective Values:
- Excellent: Diaphragmatic breathing with ease.
- Good: Mostly diaphragmatic breathing with slight chest involvement.
- Average: Equal involvement of chest and diaphragm.
- Below Average: Shallow chest breathing dominates.

9 - Awareness Test - Mindful Breathing

Instructions:
- Sit comfortably and focus on your breath for 2 minutes.
- Note how easily you can maintain focus without distractions.

Objective:
Evaluate mindfulness and concentration.

Objective Values:
- Excellent: Sustained focus for 2 minutes without distraction.
- Good: Sustained focus with occasional distraction.
- Average: Frequent distraction but able to regain focus.
- Below Average: Difficulty maintaining focus for the duration.

10 - Overall Comfort Test - Body Scan

Instructions:
- Sit or lie down and mentally scan your body from head to toe.
- Note any areas of tension or discomfort.

Objective:
Assess overall comfort and body awareness.

Objective Values:
- Excellent: No areas of tension or discomfort.
- Good: Minor tension or discomfort in specific areas.
- Average: Moderate tension or discomfort in specific areas.
- Below Average: Significant tension or discomfort in multiple areas.

These objective values provide a guideline for individuals to self-assess their fitness level based on the outcomes of each test. They can use this information to tailor their Wall Pilates journey according to their current physical capabilities and progressively improve over time.

Chapter 5: 28-Day Wall Pilates Workout Challenge

The Workout plan is based on 2 phases:
- 4 weeks to build the foundations: perfect for beginners!
- 4 weeks to increase the confidence: suitable for intermediate level.

Week 1: Foundations

This week is all about establishing a solid foundation in Wall Pilates. The emphasis is on introducing fundamental exercises, ensuring proper posture, and familiarizing beginners with the support of the wall. Workouts will be gentle yet effective, targeting core engagement and body awareness.

Key Components:
- Introduction to basic Wall Pilates poses.
- Focus on breathing techniques and mindfulness.
- Gentle exercises to activate core muscles.
- Establishing a consistent daily routine.

Objective: To build a strong foundation, improve posture, and initiate the mind-body connection.
Every exercise should be done at YOUR maximum (please consider the results of the assessment test)
The quality of the exercise is more important than the speed is always better to concentrate on the technic and with maximum concentration.
- If you are at beginner level, consider having 30 sec of exercises, then 30 sec of pause.
- If you are an intermediate, let's consider 45 sec of exercise, 15 sec of pause.
- If you don't feel tired with the above, let's 60 sec of exercise, 15 sec of pause.

In the Workout Table you will find:
- The step-by-step pictures of the exercises.
- the duration of the full exercise.
- the QR Code to see the professional Video.

It's not present the full step by step description to simplify the readability.
The suggestion, before starting the workout, is to look for the Exercise name in the Glossary, read the details, and then start the Workout, using the QR code to see the Professional Video

<table>
<tr><td colspan="4" align="center">WEEK 1: FOUNDATIONS</td></tr>
<tr><td>Day</td><td>Exercise</td><td>Duration</td><td>QR code</td></tr>
<tr>
<td rowspan="4" align="center">1</td>
<td align="center">Wall Squats 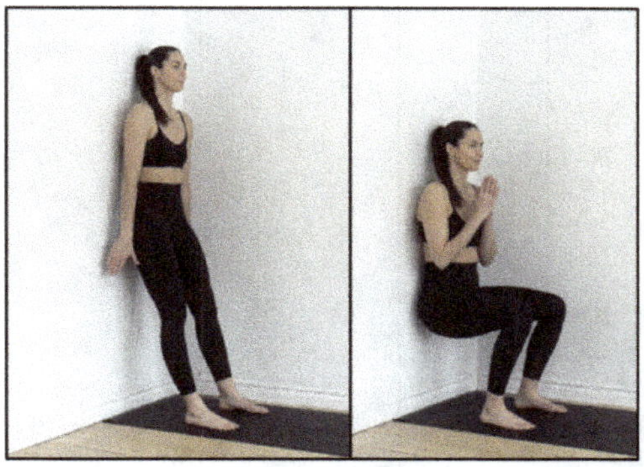</td>
<td align="center">5 mins</td>
<td rowspan="4" align="center">
https://youtu
.be/ofFYm_-
UFUM?si=itg
KakK3N5-
k5P-8</td>
</tr>
<tr>
<td align="center">Wall glute bridge 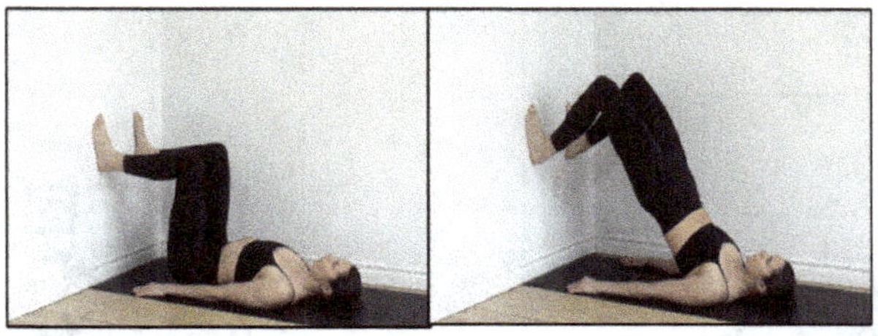</td>
<td align="center">5 min</td>
</tr>
<tr>
<td align="center">Wall Side Lunges (left) 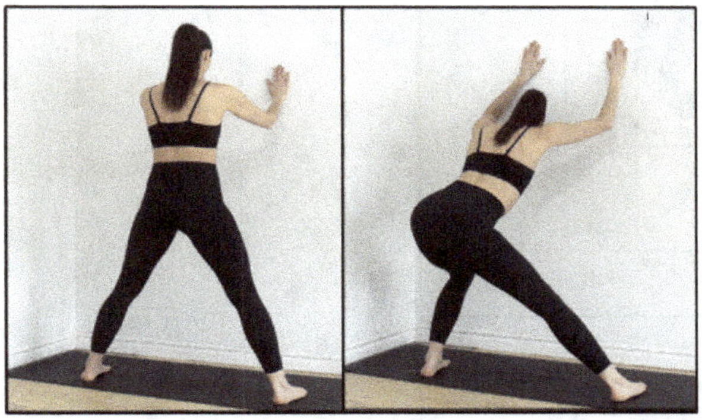</td>
<td align="center">5 min</td>
</tr>
<tr>
<td align="center">Wall Side Lunges (right) 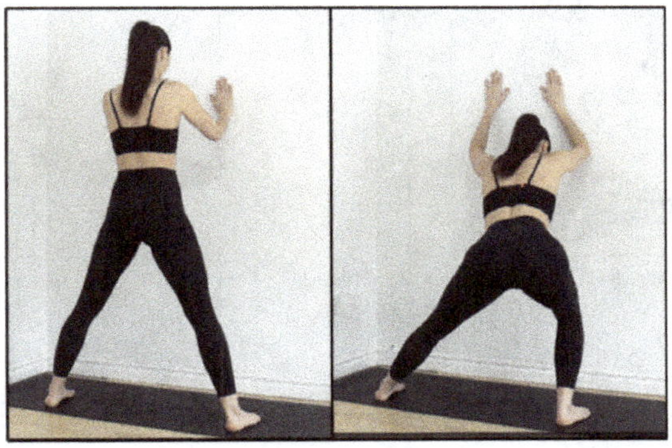</td>
<td align="center">5 min</td>
</tr>
</table>

<table>
<tr><td colspan="4" align="center">WEEK 1: FOUNDATIONS</td></tr>
<tr><td>Day</td><td align="center">Exercise</td><td>Duration</td><td>QR code</td></tr>
<tr>
<td rowspan="3" align="center">2</td>
<td align="center">Wall Push Ups 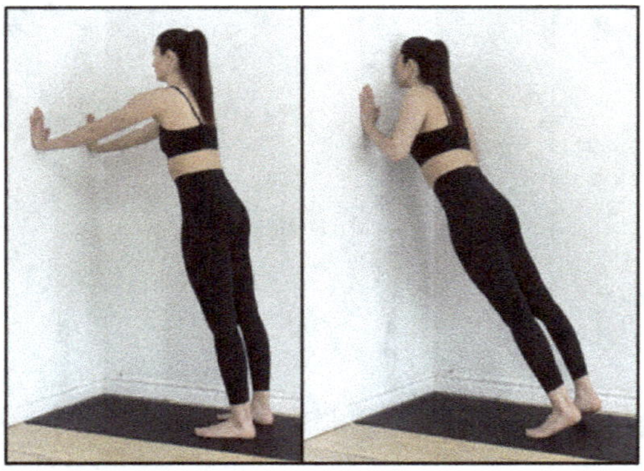</td>
<td align="center">6 min</td>
<td rowspan="3" align="center">https://youtu.be/WZq4QkfcYXg?si=h-w3-navlYX87Nws</td>
</tr>
<tr>
<td align="center">Wall Diamond Push Ups 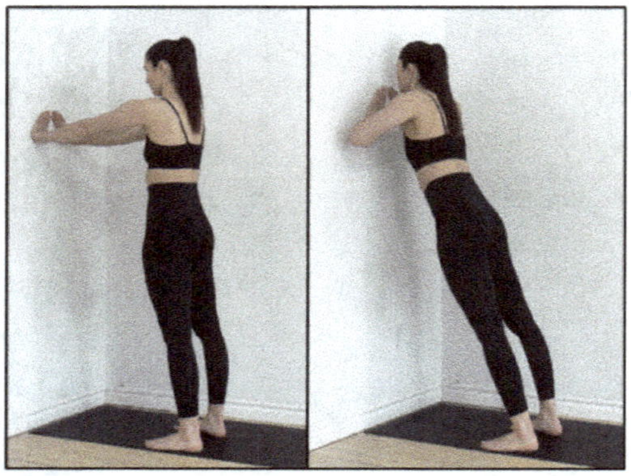</td>
<td align="center">6 min</td>
</tr>
<tr>
<td align="center">Wall Shoulder Taps 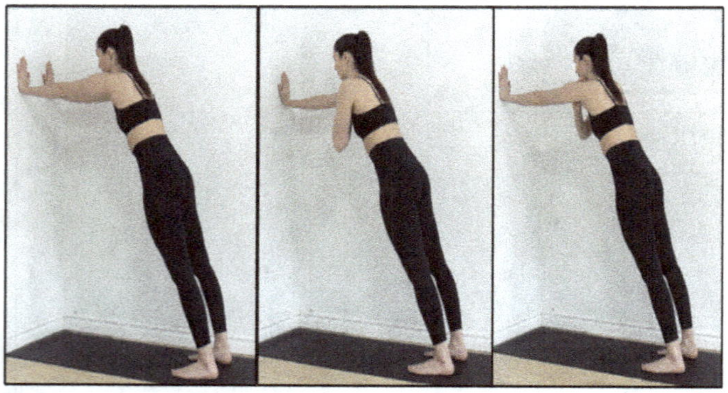</td>
<td align="center">6 min</td>
</tr>
</table>

<table>
<tr><td colspan="4" align="center">WEEK 1: FOUNDATIONS</td></tr>
<tr><td>Day</td><td align="center">Exercise</td><td>Duration</td><td>QR code</td></tr>
<tr>
<td rowspan="3">3</td>
<td align="center">Wall standing knee drives 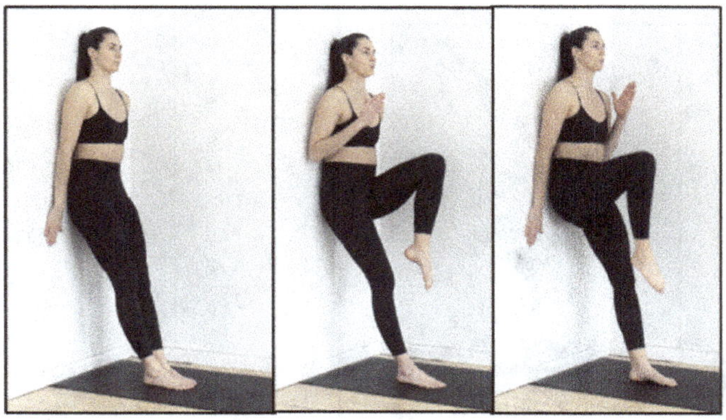</td>
<td>6 mins</td>
<td rowspan="3">https://youtu.b e/enkPZAJAuyc ?si=jrVJ_C4Mq RjfsbV3</td>
</tr>
<tr>
<td align="center">Wall Cross Body Crunches 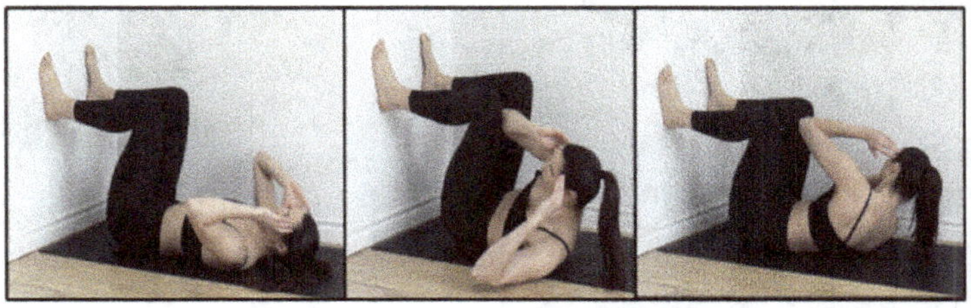</td>
<td>6 min</td>
</tr>
<tr>
<td align="center">Wall Reach Through Crunches 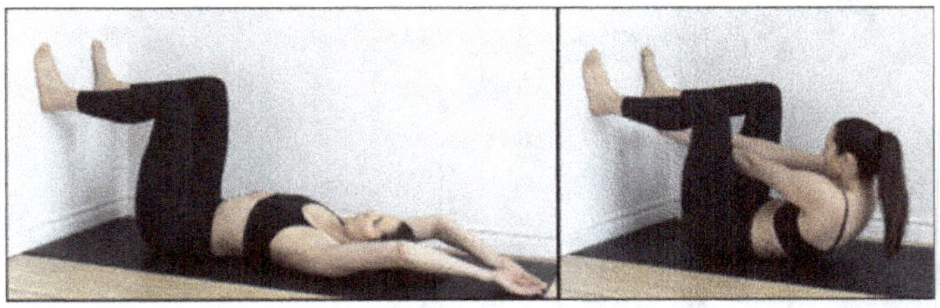</td>
<td>6 min</td>
</tr>
</table>

<table>
<tr><th colspan="4">WEEK 1: FOUNDATIONS</th></tr>
<tr><th>Day</th><th>Exercises</th><th>Duration</th><th>QR code</th></tr>
<tr>
<td rowspan="3">4</td>
<td>Wall Sit with Leg Extensions 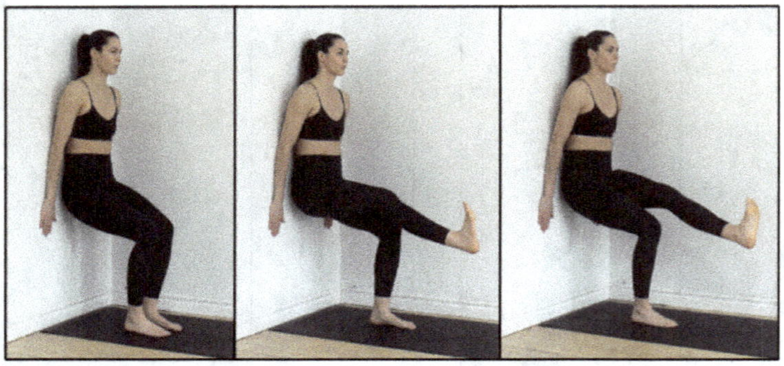</td>
<td>6 mins</td>
<td rowspan="3">https://youtu.be/yCYKnx1UqS4?si=2zq6DkOiKFfZ4dQx</td>
</tr>
<tr>
<td>Wall Glute Kickbacks (Right) 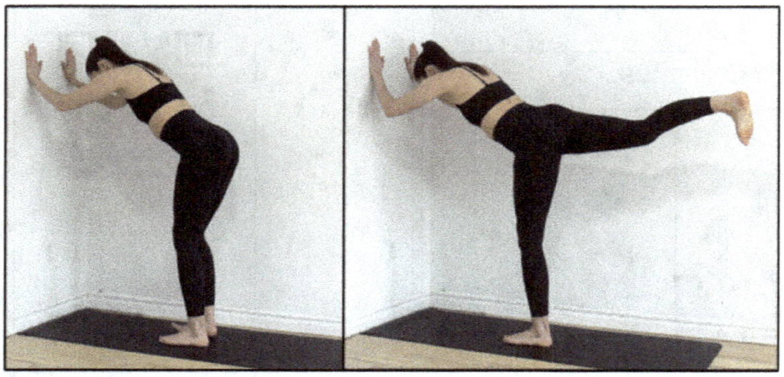</td>
<td>6 mins</td>
</tr>
<tr>
<td>Wall Glute Kickbacks (Left) 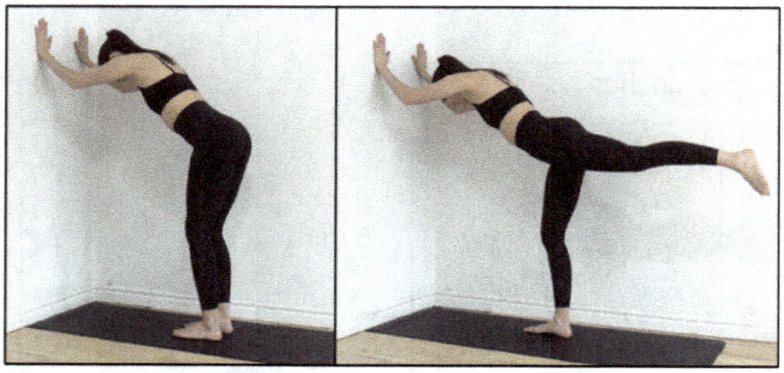</td>
<td>6 mins</td>
</tr>
</table>

<table>
<tr><td colspan="4" style="text-align:center">WEEK 1: FOUNDATIONS</td></tr>
<tr><th>Day</th><th>Exercises</th><th>Duration</th><th>QR code</th></tr>
<tr>
<td rowspan="3">5</td>
<td>Wall Tricep Press 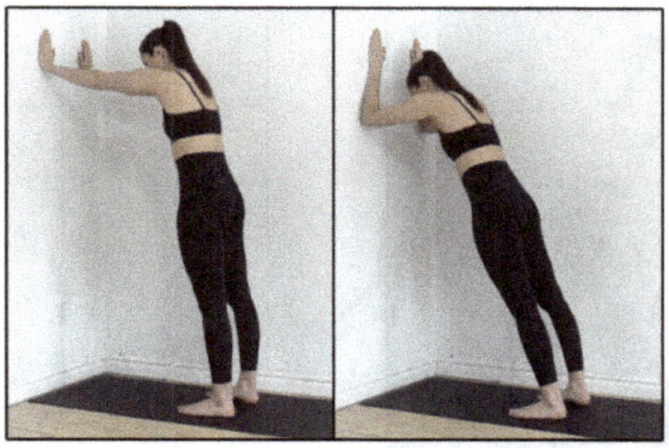</td>
<td>6 mins</td>
<td rowspan="3">https://youtu.be/fM1AVtcUGbo?si=Njjzq_izLjYlQD7y</td>
</tr>
<tr>
<td>Wall Arm Angels 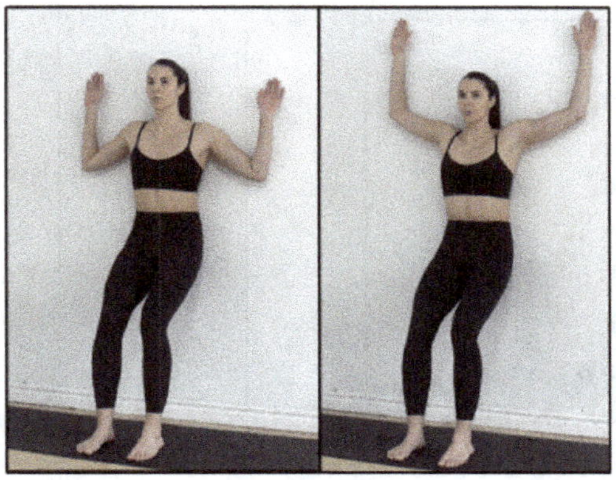</td>
<td>6 mins

6 mins</td>
</tr>
<tr>
<td>Wall Thread the Needle 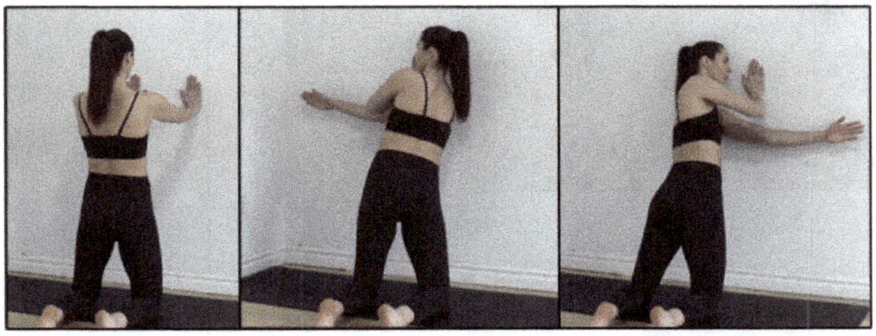</td>
<td></td>
</tr>
</table>

<table>
<tr><td colspan="4" align="center">WEEK 1: FOUNDATIONS</td></tr>
<tr><td>Day</td><td align="center">Exercises</td><td>Duration</td><td>QR code</td></tr>
<tr>
<td align="center">6</td>
<td>
Wall Plank 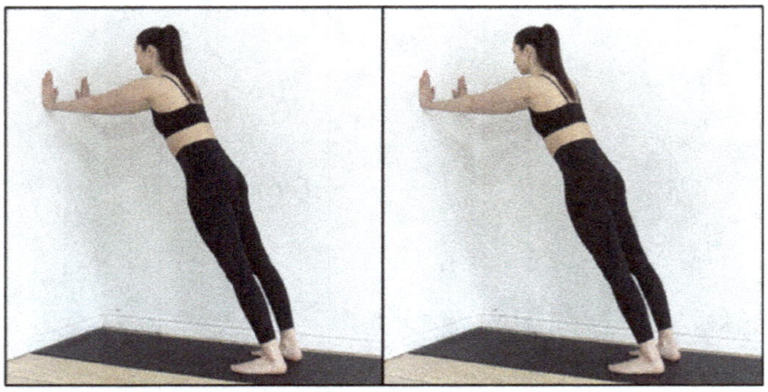

Wall Toe Touch Crunches 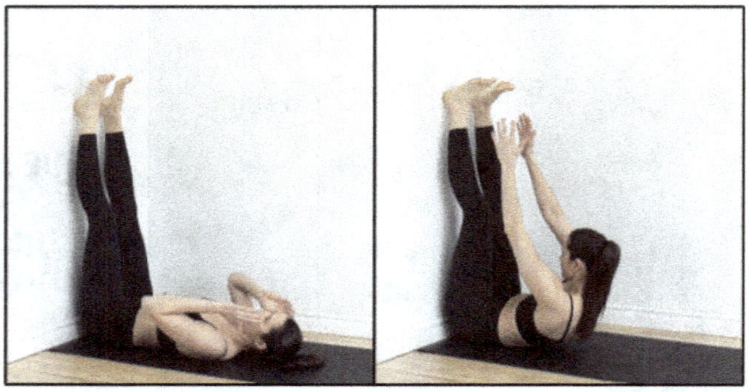

Wall Elevated Plank Side Steps 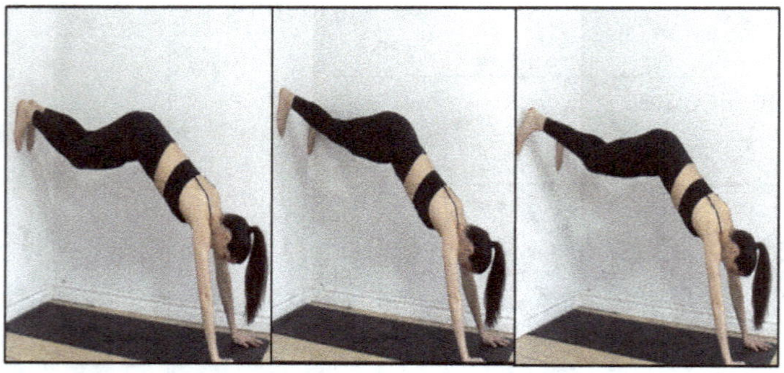
</td>
<td>6 mins

6 mins

6 mins</td>
<td>https://youtu.be/
gIi9H1j5_UM?si=1
jhzLnkjkwssbiMC</td>
</tr>
</table>

<table>
<tr><th colspan="4">WEEK 1: FOUNDATIONS</th></tr>
<tr><th>Day</th><th>Exercises</th><th>Duration</th><th>QR code</th></tr>
<tr><td rowspan="3">7</td><td>Wall Walking Glute Bridge</td><td>6 mins</td><td rowspan="3">https://youtu.be/
S0Mv1F8okxg?si=
5YtgrfCRcyiEObPX</td></tr>
<tr><td>Wall Pilates 100's</td><td>6 mins</td></tr>
<tr><td>Wall plank to pike</td><td>6 mins</td></tr>
</table>

<u>**Week 2: Building Strength**</u>

In the second week, the intensity slightly increases as participants start building strength. The workouts incorporate more challenging exercises that engage various muscle groups. The wall serves as a reliable support, allowing individuals to gradually enhance their strength and stamina.

Key Components:
- Progression to intermediate Wall Pilates poses.
- Integration of strength-building exercises.
- Emphasis on controlled movements and proper form.
- Introduction to variations for increased difficulty.

Objective: To enhance overall body strength and stamina, progressing from foundational exercises.
Every exercise should be done at YOUR maximum (please consider the results of the assessment test)
The quality of the exercise is more important than the speed is always better to concentrate on the technic and with maximum concentration.
- If you are at beginner level, consider having 30 sec of exercises, then 30 sec of pause.
- If you are an intermediate, let's consider 45 sec of exercise, 15 sec of pause.
- If you don't feel tired with the above, let's 60 sec of exercise, 15 sec of pause.

In the Workout Table you will find:
- The step-by-step pictures of the exercises.
- the duration of the full exercise.
- the QR Code to see the professional Video.

It's not present the full step by step description to simplify the readability.
The suggestion, before starting the workout, is to look for the Exercise name in the Glossary, read the details, and then start the Workout, using the QR code to see the Professional Video

WEEK 2: BUILDING STRENGHT			
Day	Exercises	Duration	QR code
1	**Wall Glute Bridge** **Wall Single Leg Glute Bridge (Right)** **Wall Single Leg Glute Bridge (Left)**	6 min 6 min 6 min	https://youtu.be/LOnndpzEgNY?si=6Izudtv_aA1J3kpn

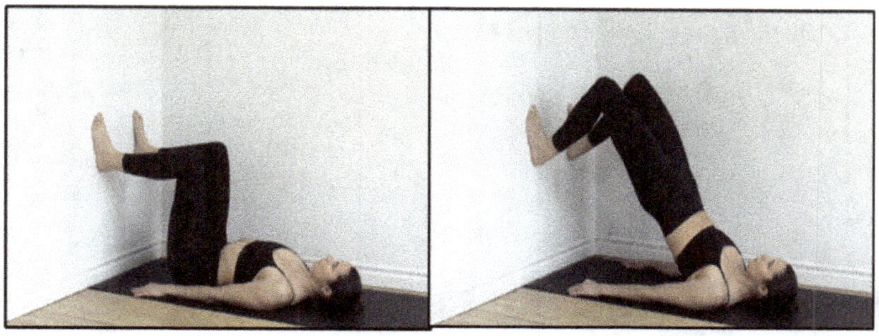

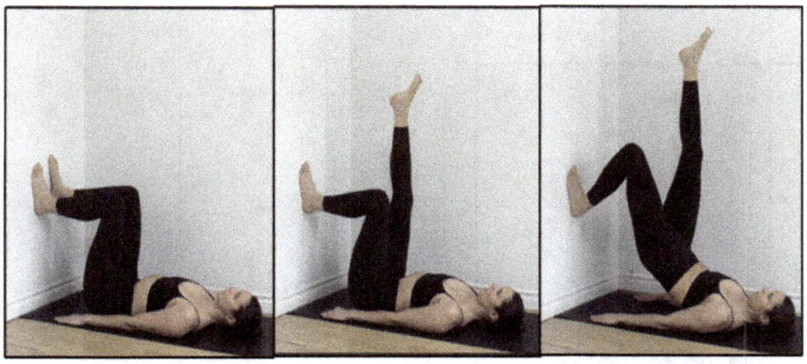

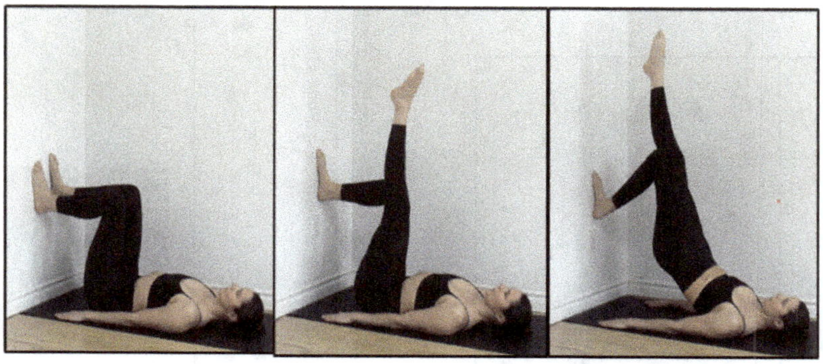

<table>
<tr><td colspan="4" align="center">WEEK 2: BUILDING STRENGHT</td></tr>
<tr><td>Day</td><td align="center">Exercises</td><td>Duratio
n</td><td>QR code</td></tr>
<tr>
<td rowspan="3" align="center">2</td>
<td align="center">Wall Push Ups</td>
<td align="center">6 min</td>
<td rowspan="3" align="center">https://youtu.
be/7SH7QAIRy
_8?si=uLaSr0q
mbUTUJEoG</td>
</tr>
<tr>
<td align="center">Wall Tricep Press</td>
<td align="center">6 min</td>
</tr>
<tr>
<td align="center">Wall Arm Angels</td>
<td align="center">6 min</td>
</tr>
</table>

<table>
<tr><th colspan="4">WEEK 2: BUILDING STRENGHT</th></tr>
<tr><th>Day</th><th>Exercises</th><th>Duration</th><th>QR code</th></tr>
<tr>
<td rowspan="3">3</td>
<td>Wall Plank 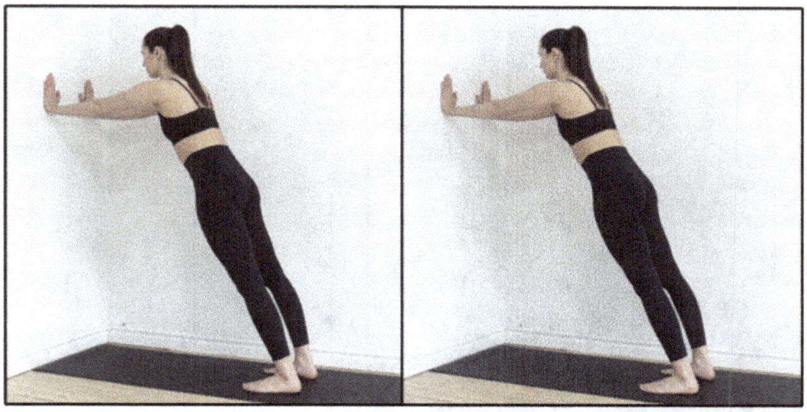</td>
<td>6 min</td>
<td rowspan="3">https://youtu.be/KY36mUnZf28?si=zohjZ0MyU4zK4675</td>
</tr>
<tr>
<td>Wall Cross Body Crunches</td>
<td>6 min</td>
</tr>
<tr>
<td>Wall Pilates 100's 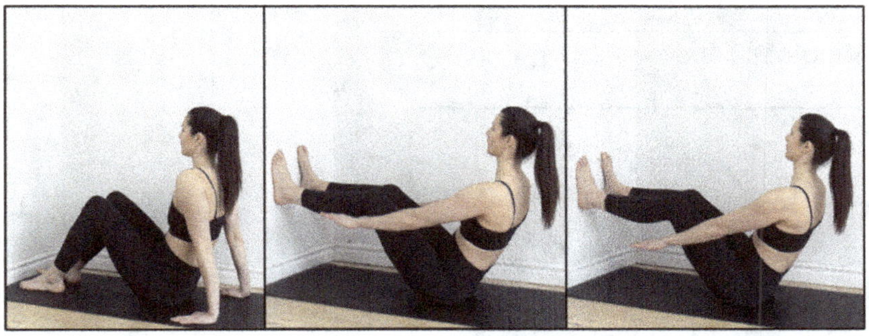</td>
<td>6 min</td>
</tr>
</table>

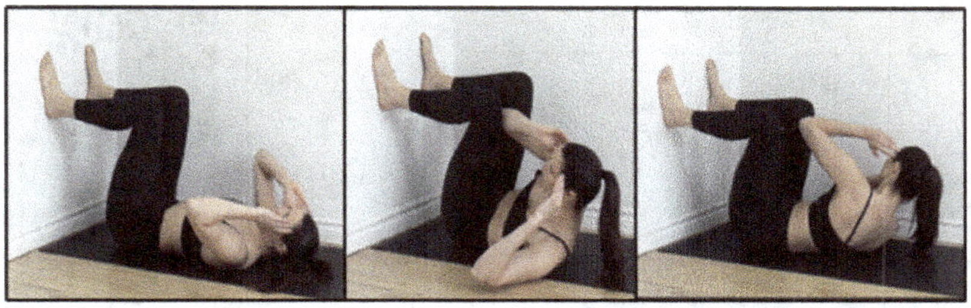

<table>
<tr><th colspan="4">WEEK 2: BUILDING STRENGHT</th></tr>
<tr><th>Day</th><th>Exercises</th><th>Duration</th><th>QR code</th></tr>
<tr>
<td rowspan="3">4</td>
<td>Wall plie squats</td>
<td>6 min</td>
<td rowspan="3">https://youtu.be/-IKIMQfUHDY?si=3Qi1SysUdIVdnR-T</td>
</tr>
<tr>
<td>Wall Diamonds</td>
<td>6 min</td>
</tr>
<tr>
<td>Wall Shoulder Taps</td>
<td>6 min</td>
</tr>
</table>

<table>
<tr><td colspan="4" align="center">WEEK 2: BUILDING STRENGHT</td></tr>
<tr><td>Day</td><td align="center">Exercises</td><td>Duratio
n</td><td>QR code</td></tr>
<tr>
<td align="center">5</td>
<td>
Wall Diamond Push Ups

Wall Commando Planks

Wall push Ups
</td>
<td>6 min

6 min

6 min</td>
<td>https://youtu.
be/K_W5nrPa
bFE?si=TaEsg3
K3NwBRHILH</td>
</tr>
</table>

<table>
<tr><th colspan="4">WEEK 2: BUILDING STRENGHT</th></tr>
<tr><th>Day</th><th>Exercises</th><th>Duration</th><th>QR code</th></tr>
<tr><td rowspan="3">6</td><td>Wall standing knee drives 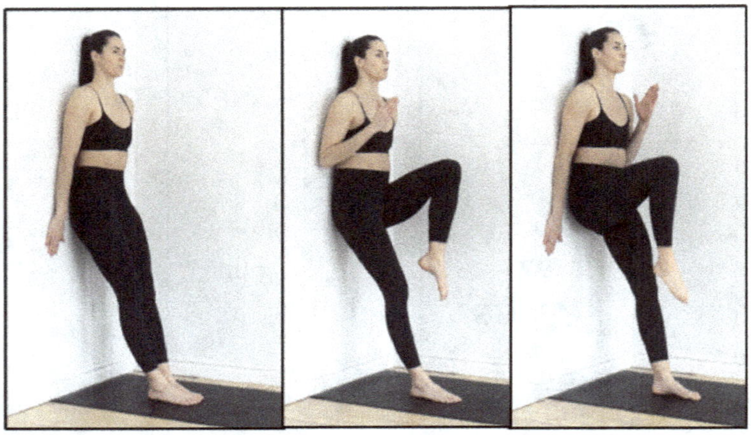</td><td>6 min</td><td rowspan="3">https://youtu.be/oOFJckCHVsA?si=gJ38pHblM6FER1fm</td></tr>
<tr><td>Wall Toe Touch Crunches 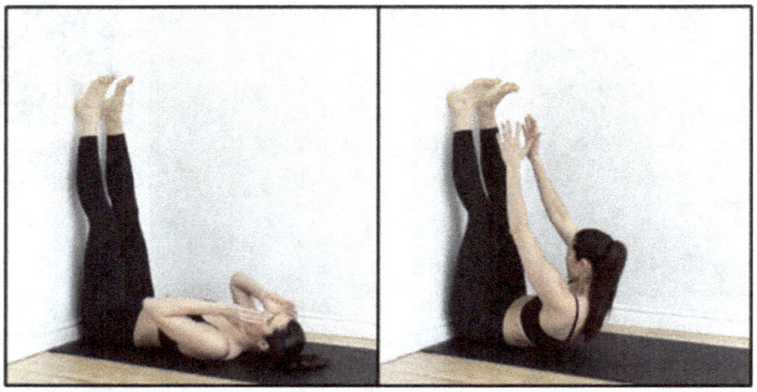</td><td>6 min</td></tr>
<tr><td>Wall Reach Through Crunches 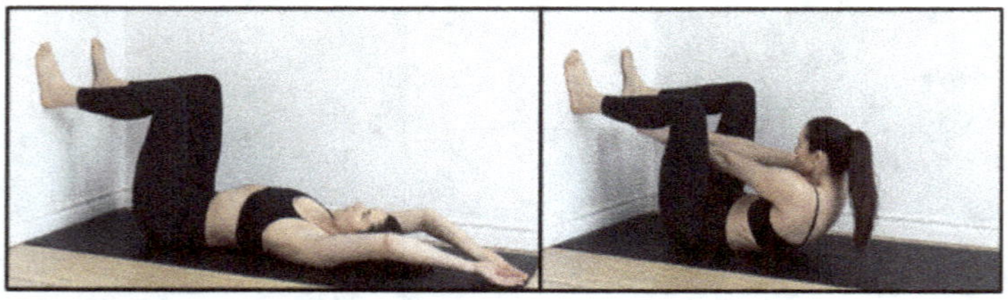</td><td>6 min</td></tr>
</table>

<table>
<tr><td colspan="4" align="center">WEEK 2: BUILDING STRENGHT</td></tr>
<tr><td>Day</td><td>Exercises</td><td>Duration</td><td>QR code</td></tr>
<tr><td rowspan="3">7</td><td>Wall Reach Through Crunches 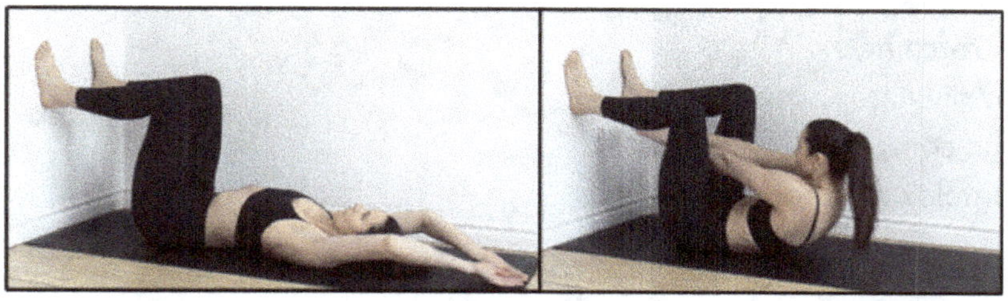</td><td>6 min</td><td rowspan="3">https://youtu.be/ykVbbljJwpU?si=ODgL9QhHj_FepW5Y</td></tr>
<tr><td>Wall plank to pike 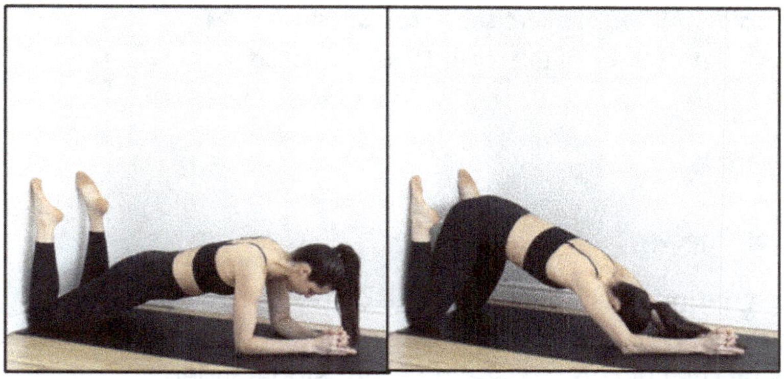</td><td>6 min</td></tr>
<tr><td>Wall Walking Glute Bridge 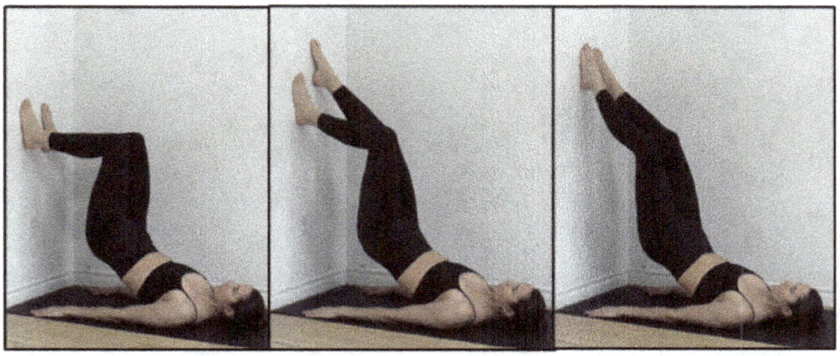</td><td>6 min</td></tr>
</table>

Week 3: Flexibility and Balance

Flexibility and balance are essential components of a well-rounded fitness routine. Week 3 focuses on stretching exercises that improve flexibility and balance. Participants will experience a variety of poses designed to increase range of motion and stability.

Key Components:
- Inclusion of dynamic and static stretching exercises.
- Integration of balance-focused Wall Pilates poses.
- Emphasis on fluid movements and controlled balance.
- Gradual introduction to more complex sequences.

Objective: To enhance flexibility, improve balance, and refine control over movements.

Every exercise should be done at YOUR maximum (please consider the results of the assessment test)

The quality of the exercise is more important than the speed is always better to concentrate on the technic and with maximum concentration.
- If you are at beginner level, consider having 30 sec of exercises, then 30 sec of pause.
- If you are an intermediate, let's consider 45 sec of exercise, 15 sec of pause.
- If you don't feel tired with the above, let's 60 sec of exercise, 15 sec of pause.

In the Workout Table you will find:
- The step-by-step pictures of the exercises.
- the duration of the full exercise.
- the QR Code to see the professional Video.

It's not present the full step by step description to simplify the readability.

The suggestion, before starting the workout, is to look for the Exercise name in the Glossary, read the details, and then start the Workout, using the QR code to see the Professional Video

WEEK 3: FLEXIBILITY AND BALANCE			
Day	Exercises	Duration	QR code
1	**Wall Side Lunges (Right)** **Wall Side Lunges (Left)** **Wall Glute Bridge**	6 min 6 min 6 min	https://youtu .be/JKRdTHA DLSY?si=gSE QlZqemkAEz FuT

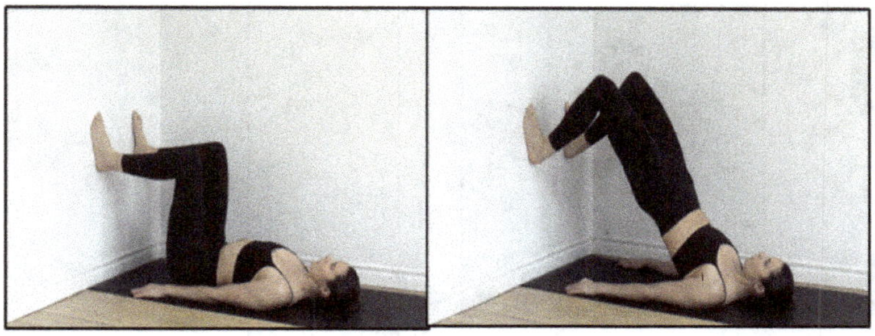

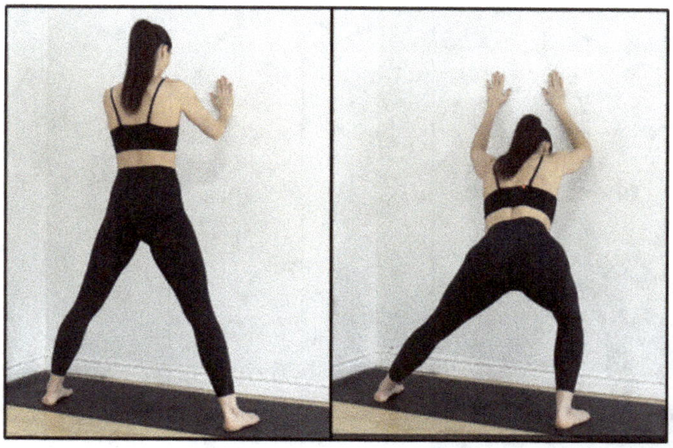

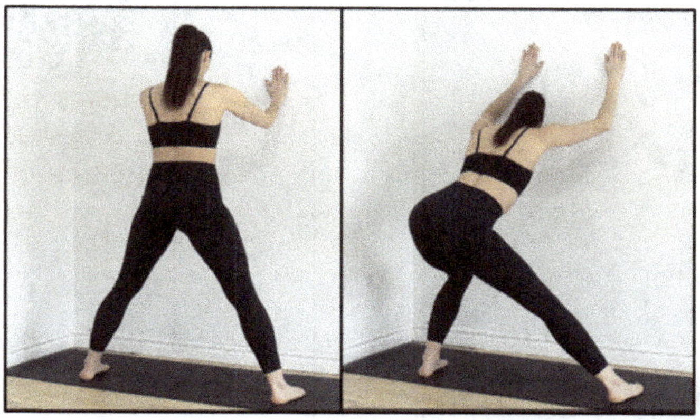

<table>
<tr><td colspan="4" align="center">WEEK 3: FLEXIBILITY AND BALANCE</td></tr>
<tr><td>Day</td><td>Exercises</td><td>Duration</td><td>QR code</td></tr>
<tr>
<td rowspan="3">2</td>
<td align="center">Wall Arm Angels 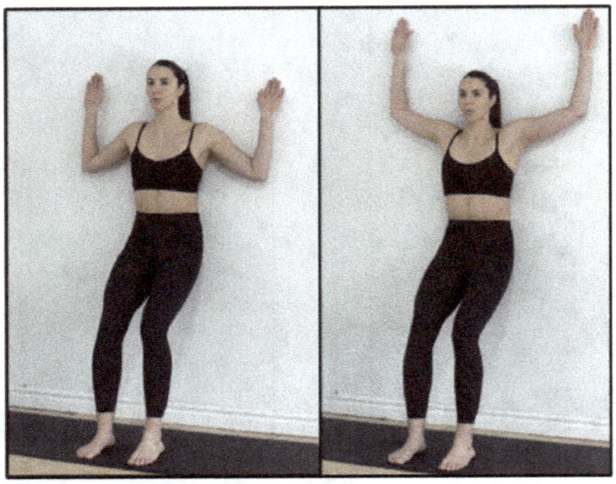</td>
<td>6 min</td>
<td rowspan="3">
https://youtu
.be/JAp8v75
wZPA?si=u68
EoqCXu4dfpI
0J</td>
</tr>
<tr>
<td align="center">Wall Arm Butterflies 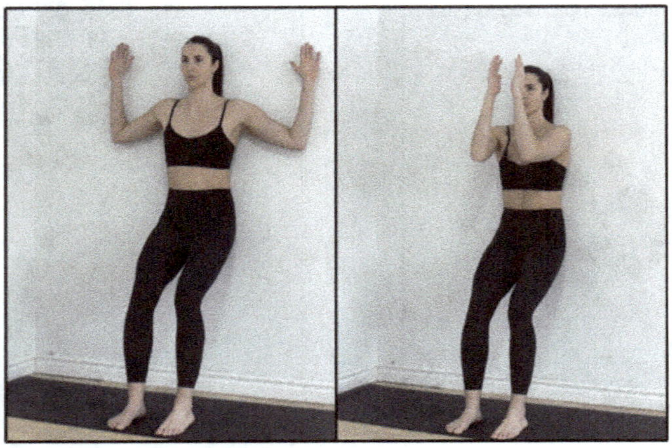</td>
<td>6 min</td>
</tr>
<tr>
<td align="center">Wall Thread the Needle 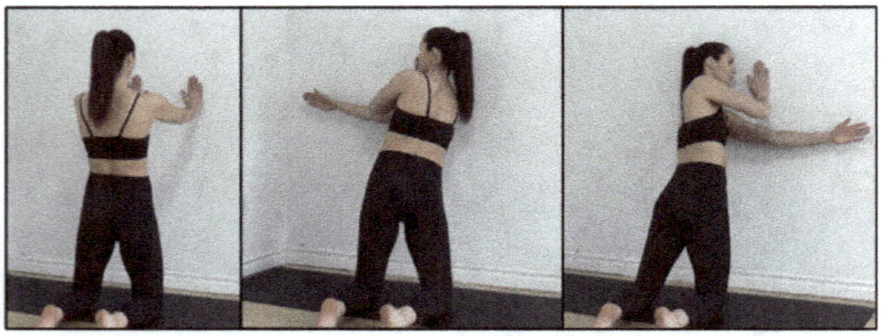</td>
<td>6 min</td>
</tr>
</table>

<table>
<tr><th colspan="4">WEEK 3: FLEXIBILITY AND BALANCE</th></tr>
<tr><th>Day</th><th>Exercises</th><th>Duration</th><th>QR code</th></tr>
<tr>
<td rowspan="3">3</td>
<td>Wall Reach Through Crunches</td>
<td>6 mins</td>
<td rowspan="3">https://youtu.be/Q0GHp0n9iDM?si=MWpCtdbSjsxzN687</td>
</tr>
<tr>
<td>Wall standing knee drives</td>
<td>6 mins</td>
</tr>
<tr>
<td>Wall Elevated Plank</td>
<td>6 mins</td>
</tr>
</table>

<table>
<tr><td colspan="4" align="center">WEEK 3: FLEXIBILITY AND BALANCE</td></tr>
<tr><td>Day</td><td align="center">Exercises</td><td>Duration</td><td>QR code</td></tr>
<tr>
<td rowspan="3">4</td>
<td align="center">Wall Squats 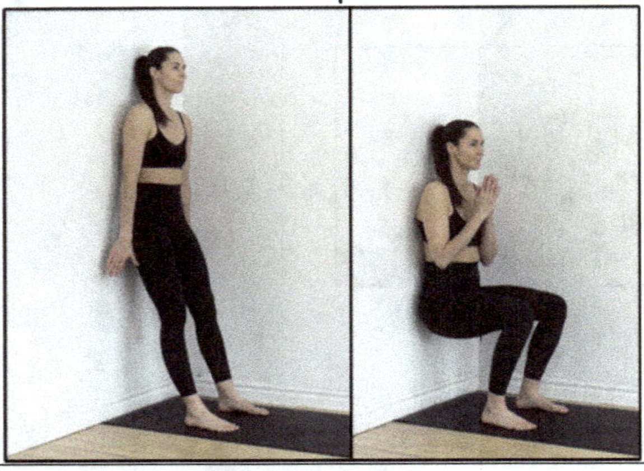</td>
<td>6 mins</td>
<td rowspan="3">https://youtu.be/xk59wKJl2Wk?si=3qVkOClP9qY0bAoe</td>
</tr>
<tr>
<td align="center">Wall Diamonds 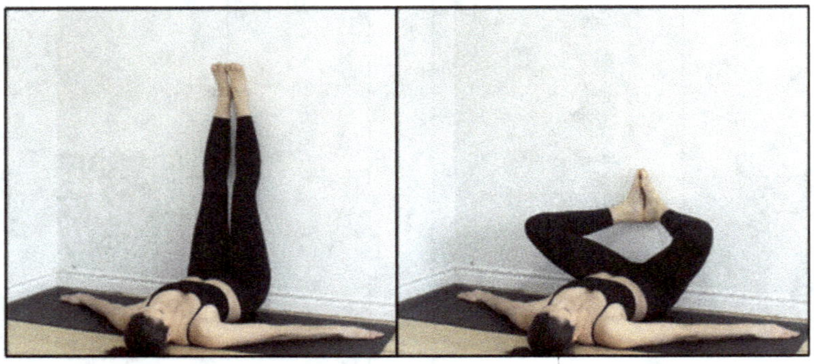</td>
<td>6 mins</td>
</tr>
<tr>
<td align="center">Wall Lying Hip Adductions 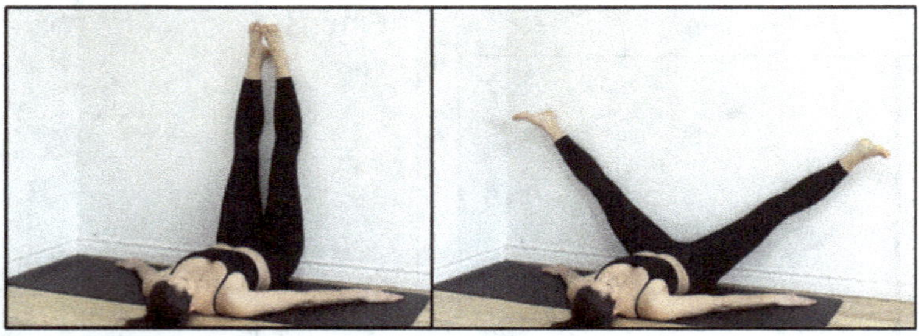</td>
<td>6 mins</td>
</tr>
</table>

WEEK 3: FLEXIBILITY AND BALANCE			
Day	Exercises	Duration	QR code
5	**Wall Push Ups** **Wall Tricep Press** **Wall Single Arm Tricep Press (Right+Left)**	6 min 6 min 6 min	https://youtu.be/kY9pFp6ZFik?si=vjoySj-lRWDK5iij

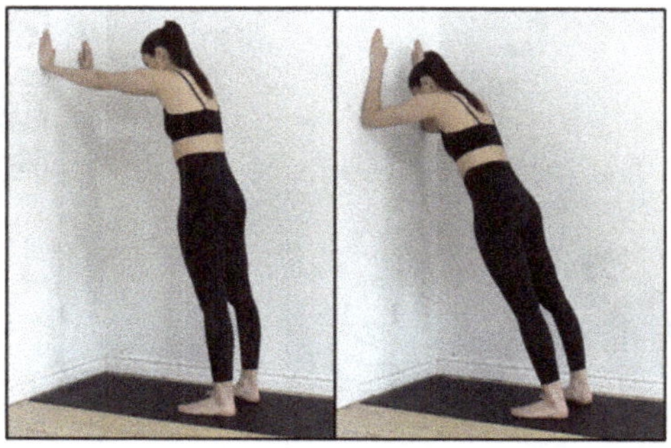

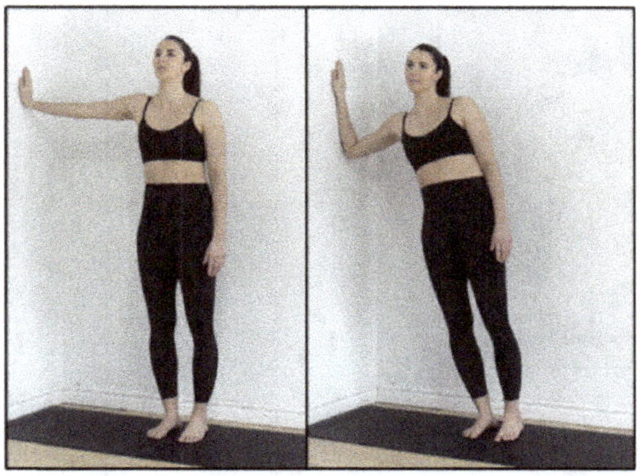

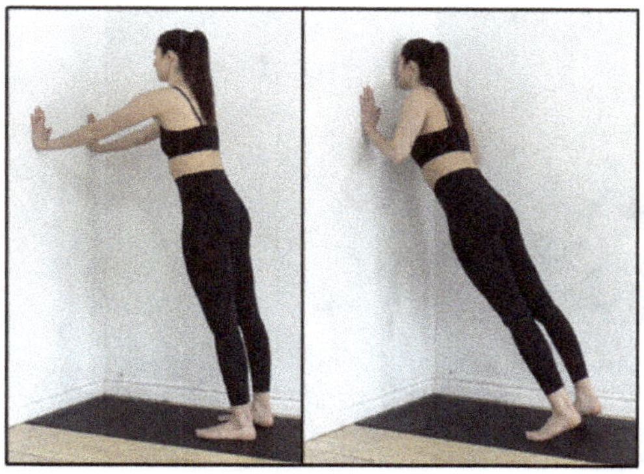

<table>
<tr><th colspan="4">WEEK 3: FLEXIBILITY AND BALANCE</th></tr>
<tr><th>Day</th><th>Exercises</th><th>Duration</th><th>QR code</th></tr>
<tr>
<td>6</td>
<td>

Wall Pilates 100's 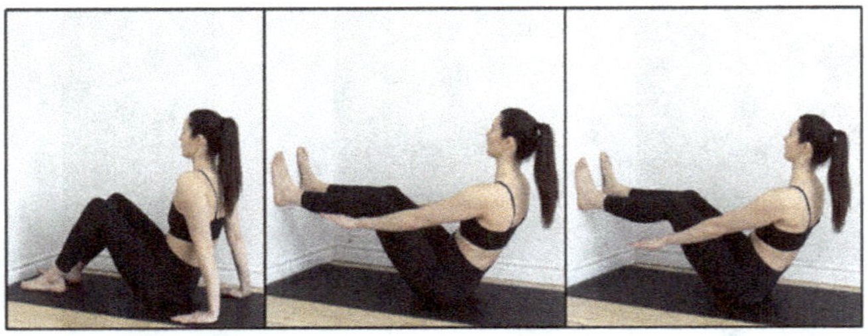

Wall plank to pike

Wall standing knee drives

</td>
<td>6 min

6 min

6 min</td>
<td>

https://youtu.be/lk13gtVCcwE?si=H2zihvSadPUKTsax

</td>
</tr>
</table>

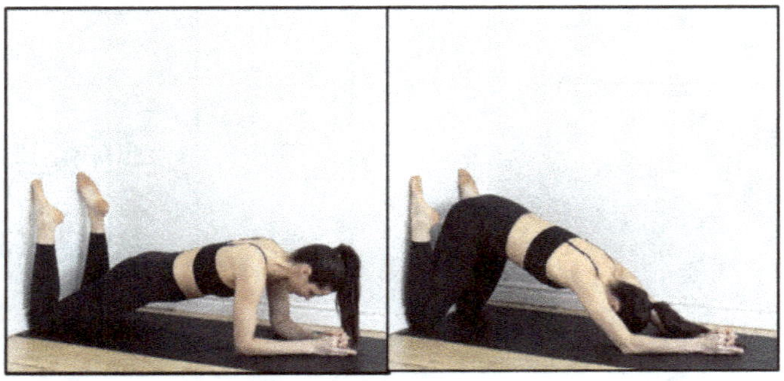

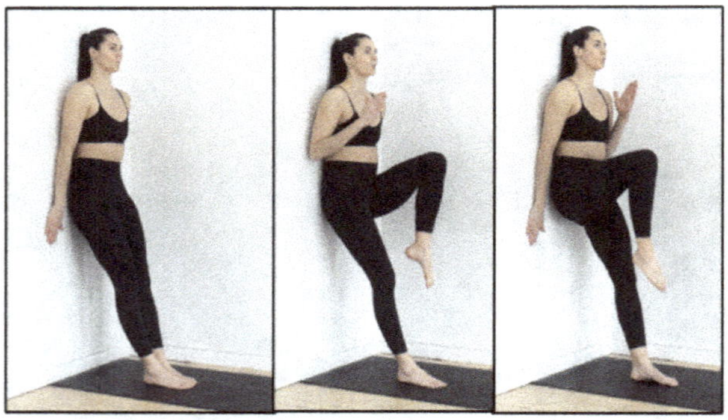

<table>
<tr><td colspan="4" align="center">WEEK 3: FLEXIBILITY AND BALANCE</td></tr>
<tr><td>Day</td><td>Exercises</td><td>Duration</td><td>QR code</td></tr>
<tr>
<td rowspan="2">7</td>
<td align="center">Wall plank to pike 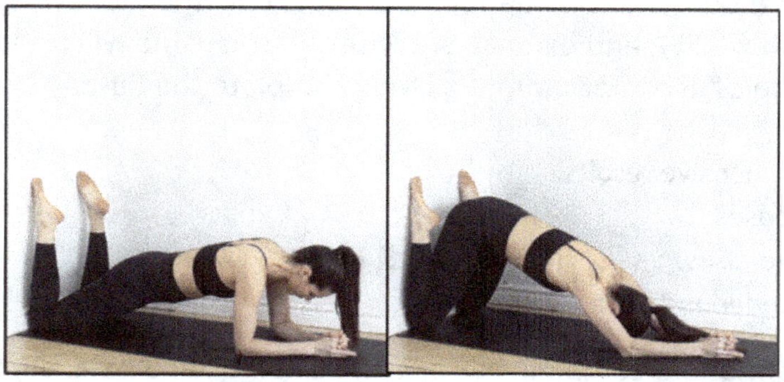</td>
<td>7 min</td>
<td rowspan="2">https://youtu
.be/envSeGC
XnYs?si=GhU
FmmFEHqQf
pfpi</td>
</tr>
<tr>
<td align="center">Wall Walking Glute Bridge 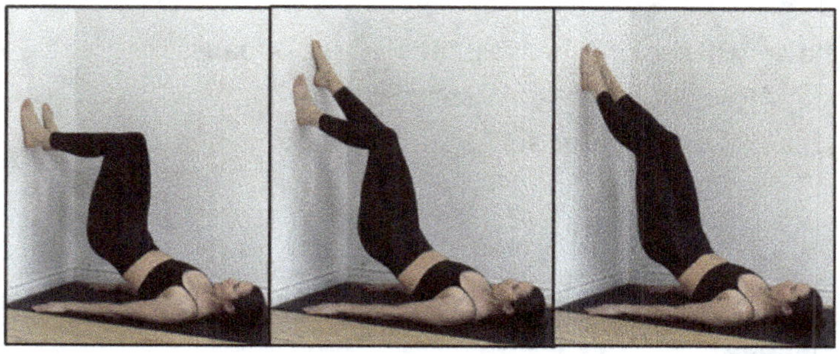</td>
<td>7 min</td>
</tr>
</table>

Week 4: Total Body Transformation

The final week is designed for a total body transformation. Workouts become more dynamic, incorporating a combination of strength, flexibility, and balance exercises. Participants will notice improvements in overall fitness and a sense of accomplishment as they complete the 28-day challenge.

Key Components:
- Full-body workout routines for comprehensive results.
- Integration of advanced Wall Pilates poses.
- Increased intensity and duration of exercises.
- Encouragement to push personal boundaries for transformation.

Objective: To achieve a total body transformation, combining strength, flexibility, and balance, and instilling a sense of accomplishment.

Every exercise should be done at YOUR maximum (please consider the results of the assessment test)

The quality of the exercise is more important than the speed is always better to concentrate on the technic and with maximum concentration.
- If you are at beginner level, consider having 30 sec of exercises, then 30 sec of pause.
- If you are an intermediate, let's consider 45 sec of exercise, 15 sec of pause.
- If you don't feel tired with the above, let's 60 sec of exercise, 15 sec of pause.

In the Workout Table you will find:
- The step-by-step pictures of the exercises.
- the duration of the full exercise.
- the QR Code to see the professional Video.

It's not present the full step by step description to simplify the readability.

The suggestion, before starting the workout, is to look for the Exercise name in the Glossary, read the details, and then start the Workout, using the QR code to see the Professional Video

<table>
<tr><th colspan="4">WEEK 4: Total Body Transformation</th></tr>
<tr><th>Day</th><th>Exercises</th><th>Duration</th><th>QR code</th></tr>
<tr><td rowspan="3">1</td><td>

Wall Glute Bridge

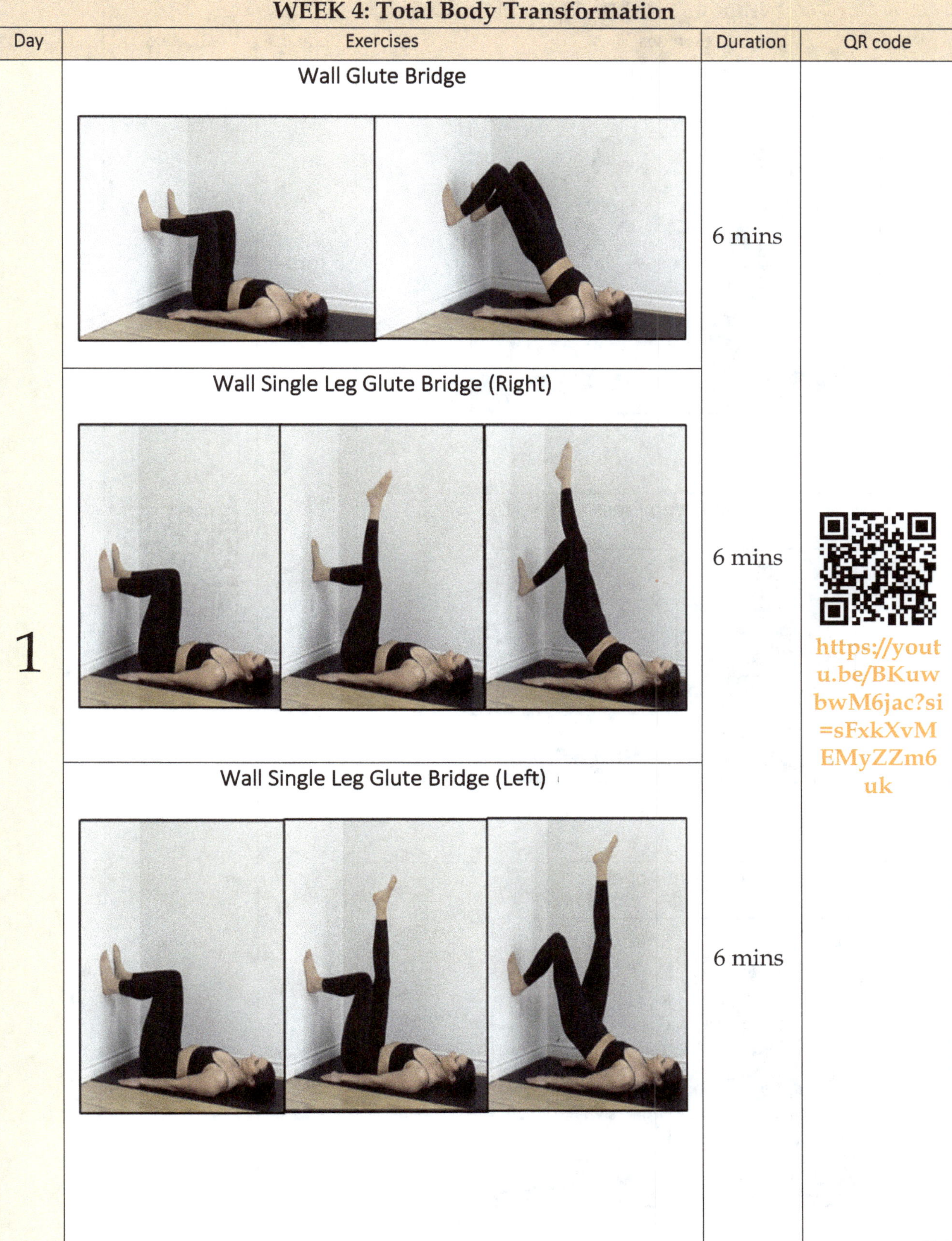

Wall Single Leg Glute Bridge (Right)

Wall Single Leg Glute Bridge (Left)

</td><td>6 mins

6 mins

6 mins</td><td>

https://youtu.be/BKuwbwM6jac?si=sFxkXvMEMyZZm6uk

</td></tr>
</table>

<table>
<tr><td colspan="4" align="center">WEEK 4: Total Body Transformation</td></tr>
<tr><td>Day</td><td align="center">Exercises</td><td>Duration</td><td>QR code</td></tr>
<tr>
<td rowspan="3">2</td>
<td align="center">Wall Push Ups</td>
<td>6 mins</td>
<td rowspan="3">https://youtu.be/REvzM-obeEo?si=cA5HhZIaqfaIVe4s</td>
</tr>
<tr>
<td align="center">Wall Tricep Press</td>
<td>6 mins</td>
</tr>
<tr>
<td align="center">Wall Arm Angels</td>
<td>6 mins</td>
</tr>
</table>

<table>
<tr><td colspan="4" align="center">WEEK 4: Total Body Transformation</td></tr>
<tr><td>Day</td><td>Exercises</td><td>Duration</td><td>QR code</td></tr>
</table>

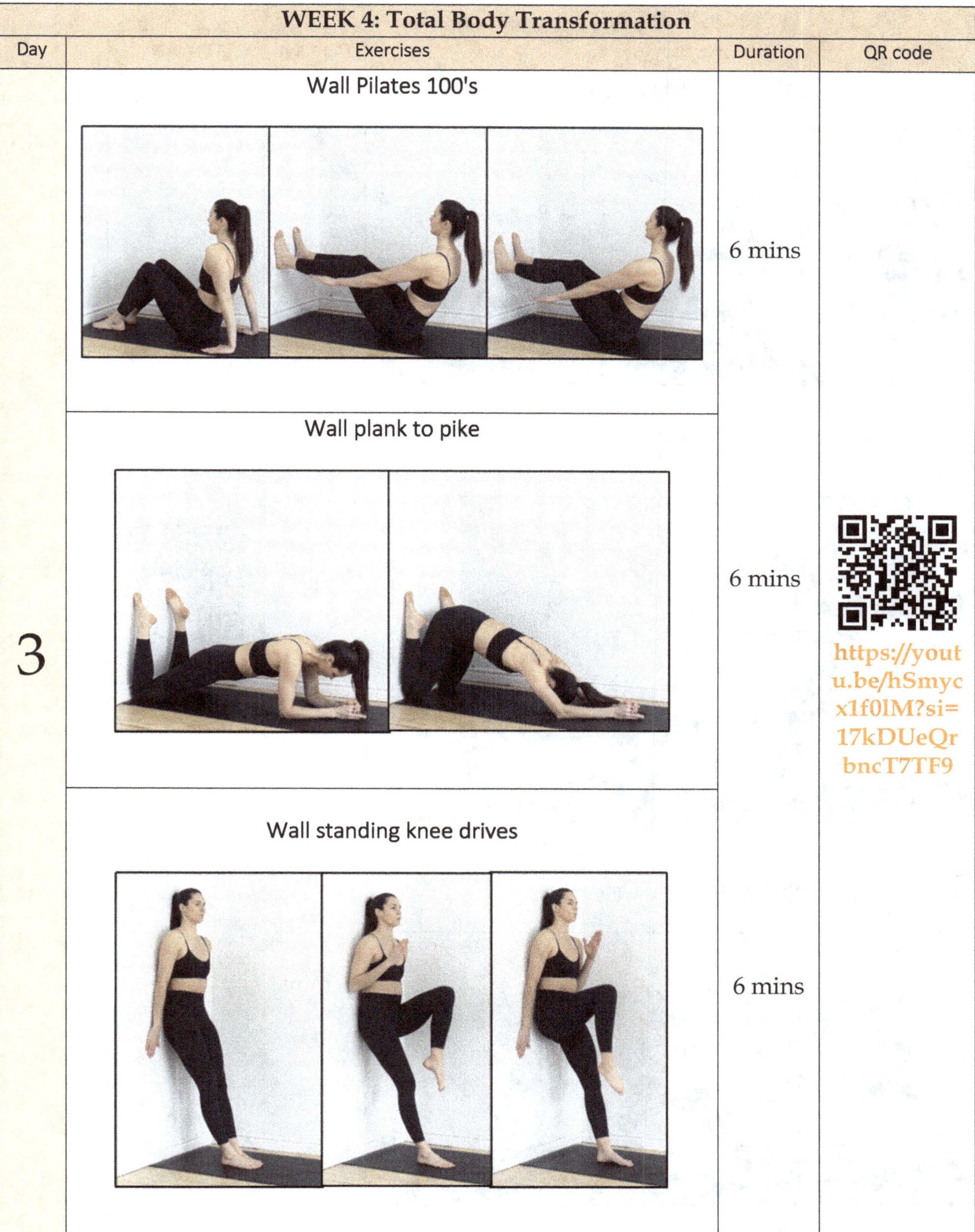

Wall Pilates 100's — 6 mins

Wall plank to pike — 6 mins

Wall standing knee drives — 6 mins

Day: 3

QR code: https://youtu.be/hSmycx1f0lM?si=17kDUeQrbncT7TF9

WEEK 4: Total Body Transformation			
Day	Exercises	Duration	QR code
4	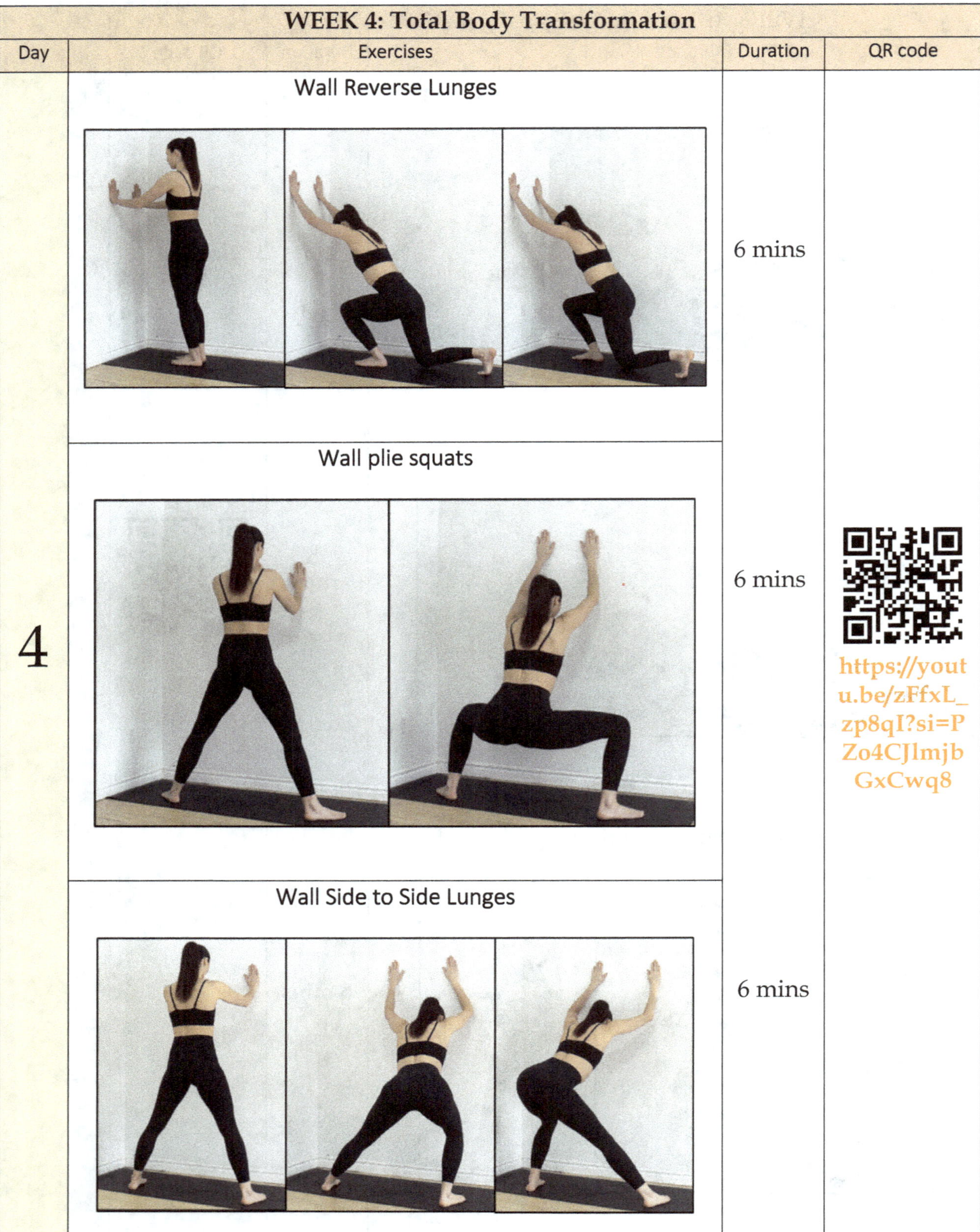 Wall Reverse Lunges Wall plie squats Wall Side to Side Lunges	6 mins 6 mins 6 mins	https://youtu.be/zFfxL_zp8qI?si=PZo4CJlmjbGxCwq8

<table>
<tr><th colspan="4">WEEK 4: Total Body Transformation</th></tr>
<tr><th>Day</th><th>Exercises</th><th>Duration</th><th>QR code</th></tr>
<tr>
<td rowspan="3">5</td>
<td>Wall Diamond Push Ups 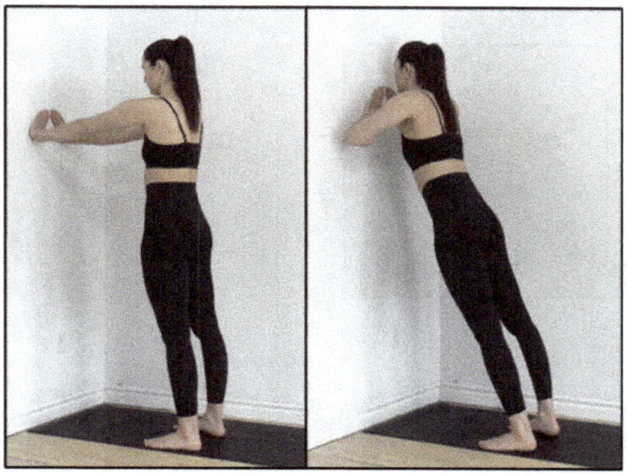</td>
<td>6 mins</td>
<td rowspan="3">https://yout
u.be/TY_tPf
Seth4?si=x
nfv_BP6Ak
ARu7I6</td>
</tr>
<tr>
<td>Wall Thread the Needle 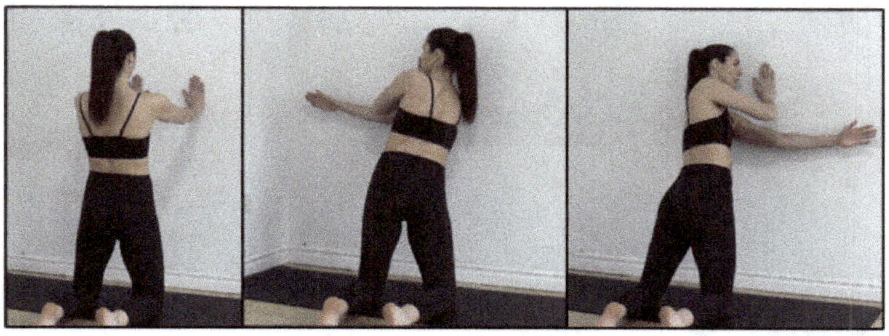</td>
<td>6 mins</td>
</tr>
<tr>
<td>Wall Arm Butterflies 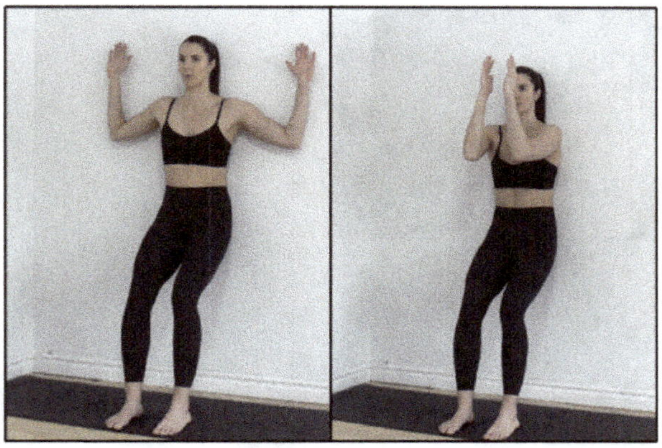</td>
<td>6 mins</td>
</tr>
</table>

<table>
<tr><th colspan="4">WEEK 4: Total Body Transformation</th></tr>
<tr><th>Day</th><th>Exercises</th><th>Duration</th><th>QR code</th></tr>
<tr>
<td>6</td>
<td>

Wall Cross Body Crunches

Wall Reach Through Crunches

Wall Pilates 100's

</td>
<td>

6 mins

6 mins

6 mins

</td>
<td>

https://youtu.be/WSW6mNEIN38?si=jgWbbeC76nihEd1w

</td>
</tr>
</table>

<table>
<tr><th colspan="4">WEEK 4: Total Body Transformation</th></tr>
<tr><th>Day</th><th>Exercises</th><th>Duration</th><th>QR code</th></tr>
</table>

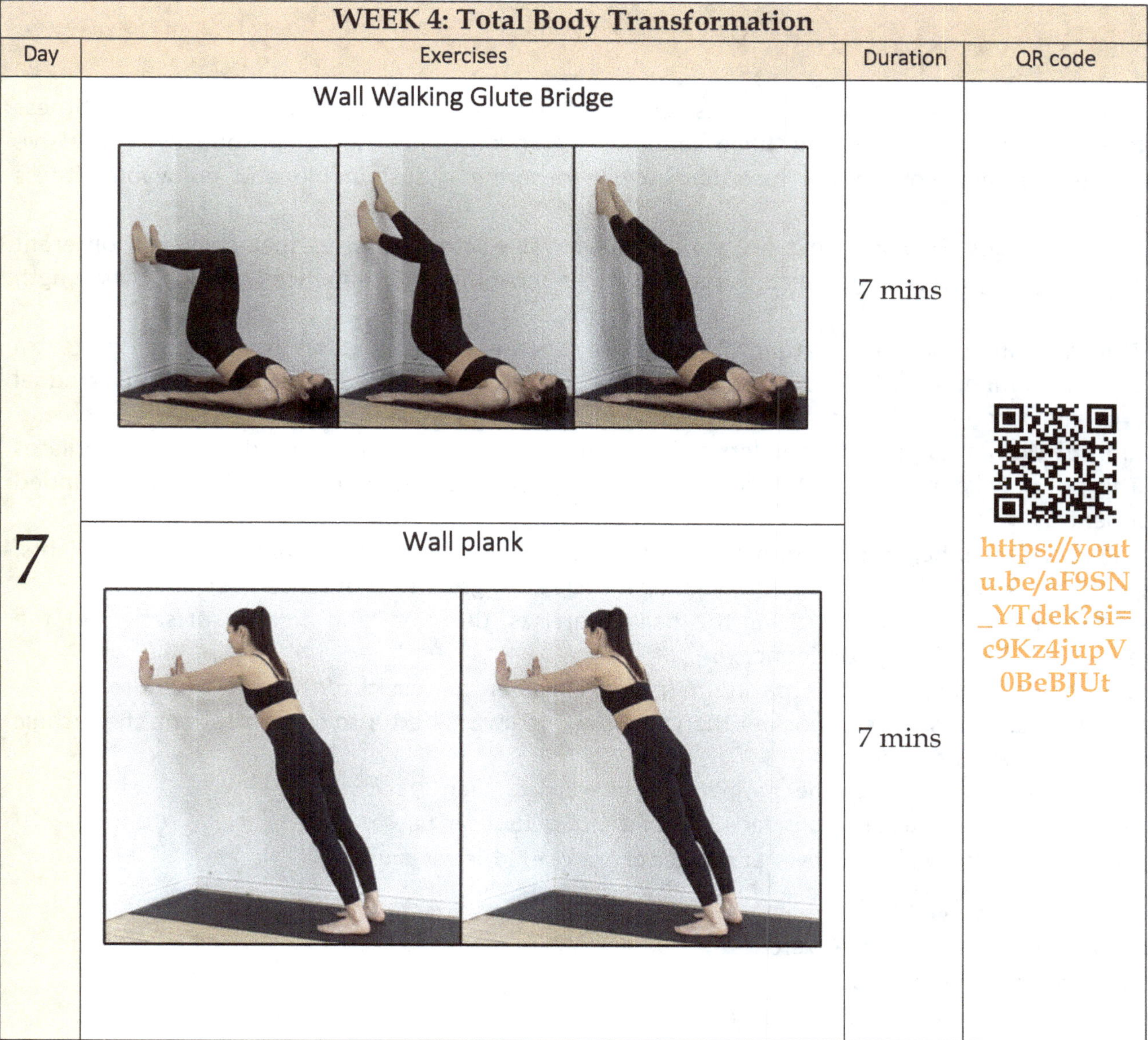

Wall Walking Glute Bridge — 7 mins

Wall plank — 7 mins

Day: 7

Chapter 6: Increasing Confidence Post 28-Day Routine

After completing the 28-day wall Pilates routine, you've laid a strong foundation for your fitness journey. Now, it's time to progress and build confidence gradually. This chapter introduces progressive routines tailored to take you to the next level while ensuring a sustainable and enjoyable fitness experience.

Integration of Advanced Exercises: explore variations of wall Pilates exercises that challenge different muscle groups. As you grow stronger, incorporate advanced movements to enhance overall body strength and flexibility.

Extended Duration: increase the duration of your daily sessions gradually. Start by adding a few extra minutes to your routine, allowing your body to adapt to extended periods of exercise. This gradual approach prevents burnout and boosts confidence in your ability to sustain longer workouts.

Diversification of Workouts: introduce diversity into your routine by incorporating different wall Pilates exercises. This not only keeps things interesting but also targets various muscle groups for a well-rounded fitness experience.

Incorporating Resistance: begin incorporating light resistance, such as resistance bands or small weights, to intensify your workouts. This step helps in building muscle strength and endurance over time.

Below is a consolidated table summarizing the daily exercises, duration, and amount of series for the Progressive Routines for Building Confidence.

Every exercise should be done at YOUR maximum (please consider the results of the assessment test)

The quality of the exercise is more important than the speed is always better to concentrate on the technic and with maximum concentration.

- If you are at beginner level, consider having 30 sec of exercises, then 30 sec of pause.
- If you are an intermediate, let's consider 45 sec of exercise, 15 sec of pause.
- If you don't feel tired with the above, let's 60 sec of exercise, 15 sec of pause.

In the Workout Table you will find:
- The step-by-step pictures of the exercises.
- the duration of the full exercise.
- the QR Code to see the professional Video.

It's not present the full step by step description to simplify the readability.

The suggestion, before starting the workout, is to look for the Exercise name in the Glossary, read the details, and then start the Workout, using the QR code to see the Professional Video

Day	Exercises	Duration	QR code
1	**Wall Pilates 100's** 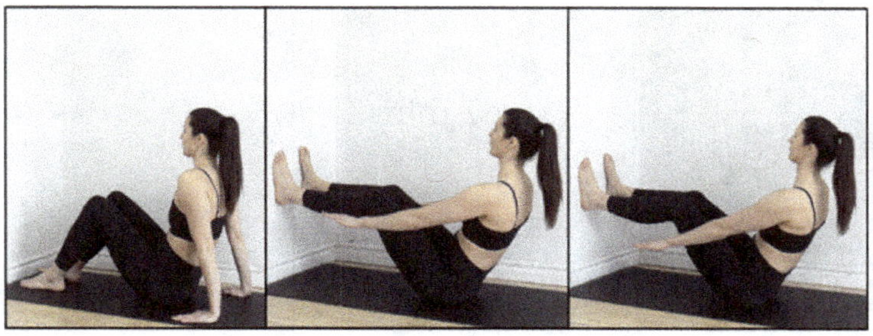	7 mins	https://youtu.be/awSuPYMMxIk?si=ZPrRE6SWAPUTl6zZ
	Wall Shoulder Taps 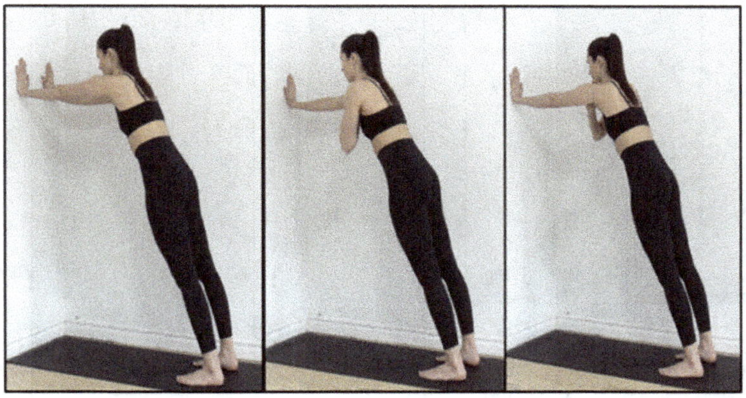	7 mins	
	Wall Push Ups 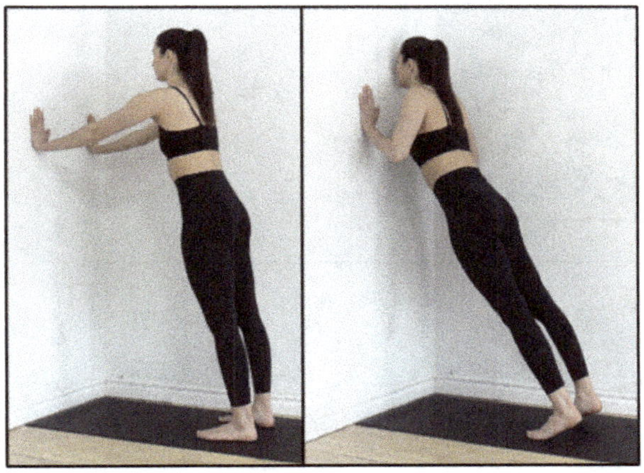	7 mins	

<table>
<tr><th colspan="4">WEEK 5: PROGRESSIVE ROUTINE 1/2</th></tr>
<tr><th>Day</th><th>Exercises</th><th>Duration</th><th>QR code</th></tr>
<tr><td rowspan="3">2</td><td>Wall Squats 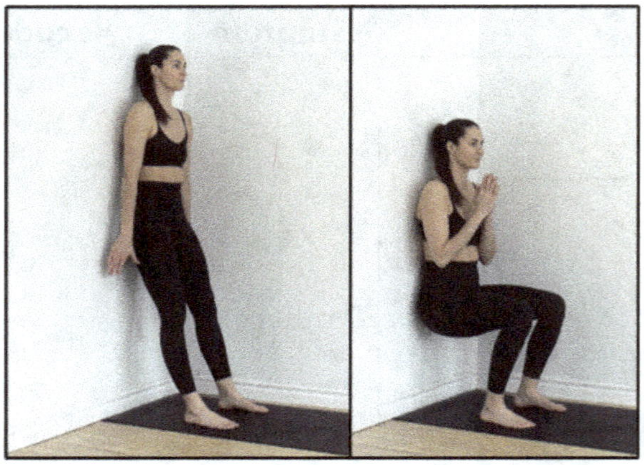</td><td>7 mins</td><td rowspan="3">https://youtu.be/Dl9mnO5I4nM?si=r15TzoCaSoe1euFV</td></tr>
<tr><td>Wall Side to Side Lunges 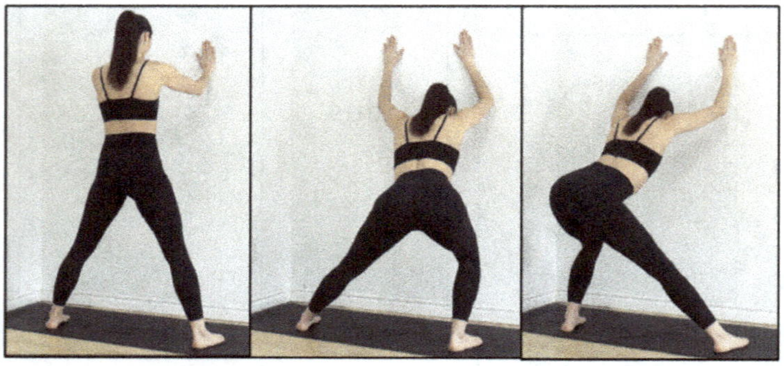</td><td>7 mins</td></tr>
<tr><td>Wall reverse Lunges 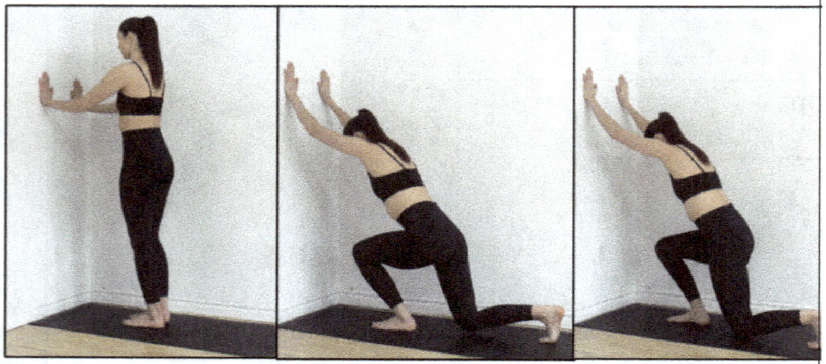</td><td>7 mins</td></tr>
</table>

<table>
<tr><td colspan="4" align="center">WEEK 5: PROGRESSIVE ROUTINE 1/2</td></tr>
<tr><td>Day</td><td align="center">Exercises</td><td>Duration</td><td>QR code</td></tr>
<tr>
<td rowspan="3" align="center">3</td>
<td align="center">Wall Reach Through Crunches</td>
<td>7 mins</td>
<td rowspan="3">https://youtu
.be/jKi98Mo
Q-
AY?si=PdGi
wIjji798I2XS</td>
</tr>
<tr>
<td align="center">Wall Pilates 100's</td>
<td>7 mins</td>
</tr>
<tr>
<td align="center">Wall plank</td>
<td>7 mins</td>
</tr>
</table>

Day	Exercises	Duration	QR code
4	**Wall Push Ups** **Wall Triceps Press** **Wall Arm Angels**	7 mins 7 mins 7 mins	https://youtu.be/b6YGAPKb1J0?si=O7HDgc5DHR0xQ5Jl

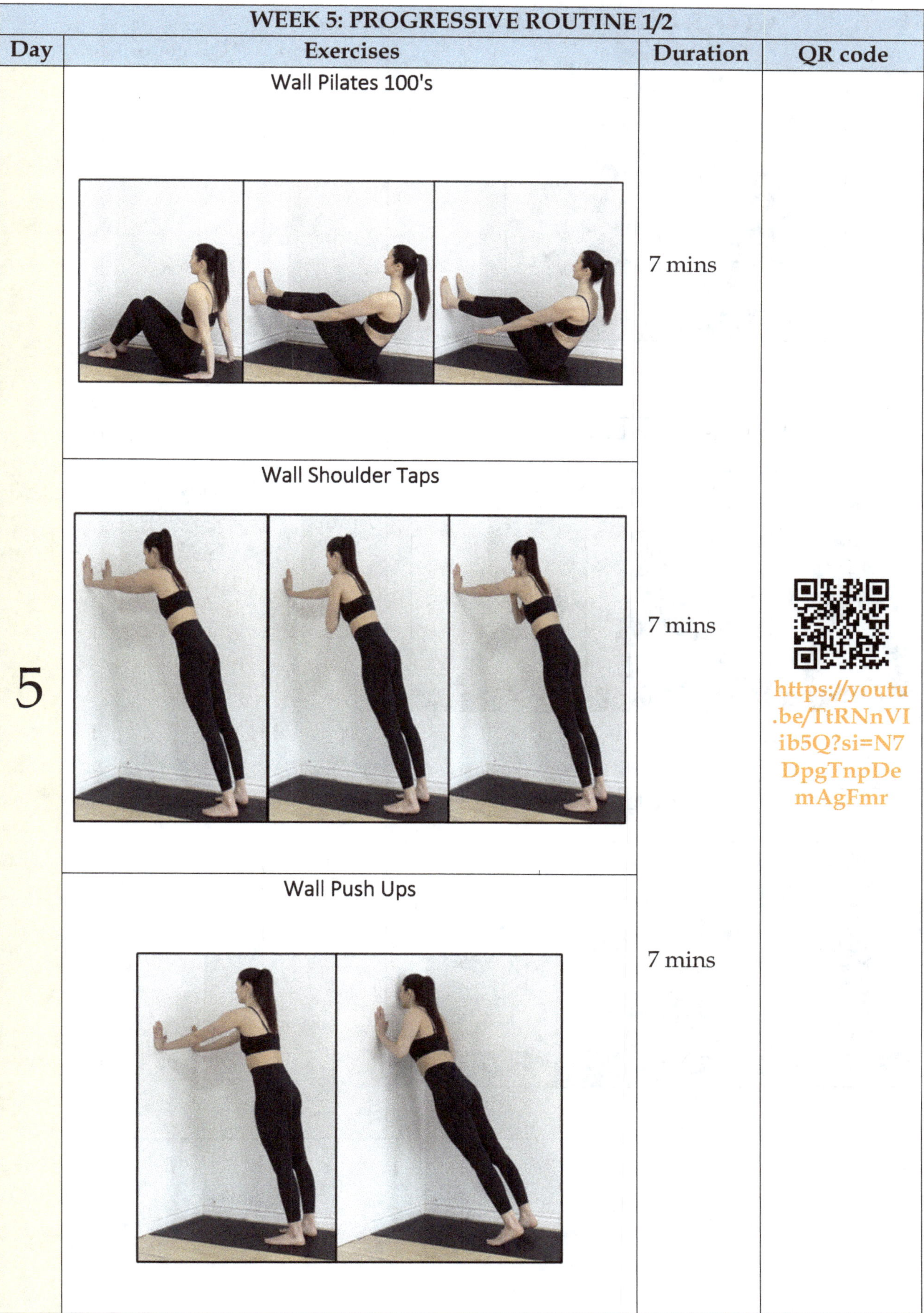

<table>
<tr><th colspan="4">WEEK 5: PROGRESSIVE ROUTINE 1/2</th></tr>
<tr><th>Day</th><th>Exercises</th><th>Duration</th><th>QR code</th></tr>
<tr><td rowspan="3">5</td><td>Wall Pilates 100's</td><td>7 mins</td><td rowspan="3"></td></tr>
<tr><td>Wall Shoulder Taps</td><td>7 mins</td></tr>
<tr><td>Wall Push Ups</td><td>7 mins</td></tr>
</table>

<table>
<tr><th colspan="4">WEEK 5: PROGRESSIVE ROUTINE 1/2</th></tr>
<tr><th>Day</th><th>Exercises</th><th>Duration</th><th>QR code</th></tr>
<tr><td rowspan="3">6</td><td>Wall Squats 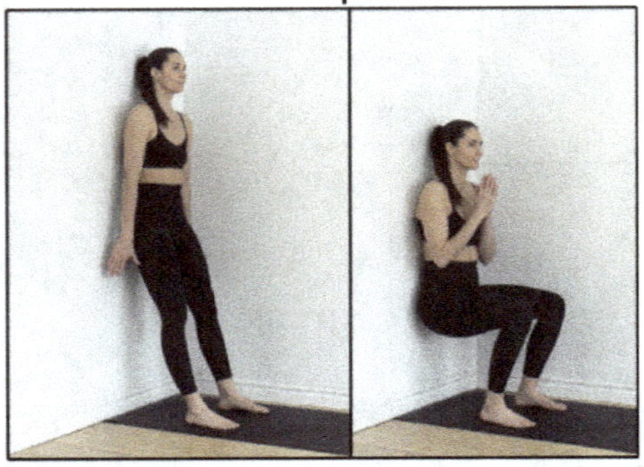</td><td>7 mins</td><td rowspan="3">https://youtu.be/Jzb1w22Y8wI?si=dTqrqC5OfApk5Zgl</td></tr>
<tr><td>Wall Side to Side Lunges 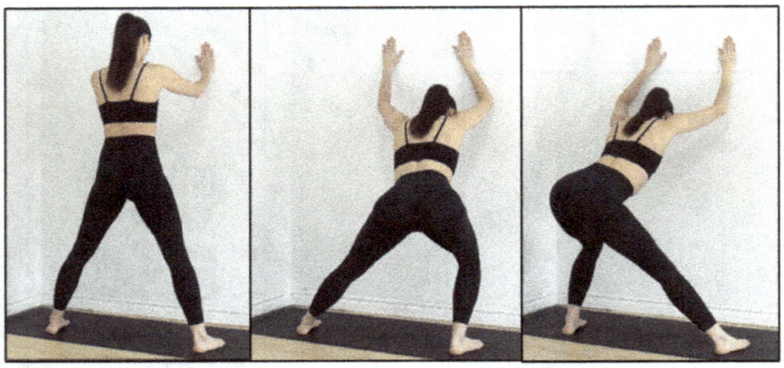</td><td>7 mins</td></tr>
<tr><td>Wall reverse lunges 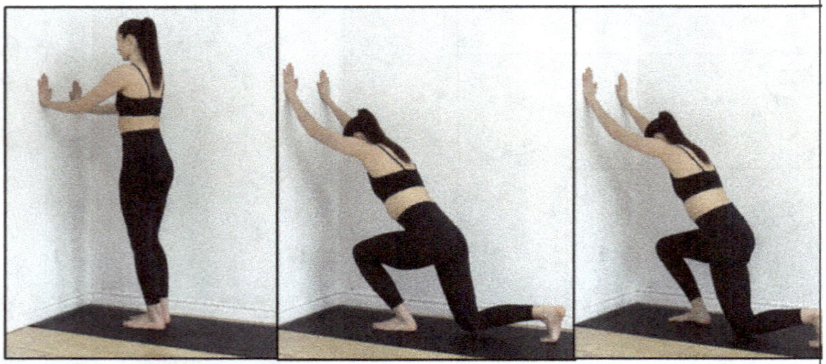</td><td>7 mins</td></tr>
</table>

<table>
<tr><th colspan="4">WEEK 5: PROGRESSIVE ROUTINE 1/2</th></tr>
<tr><th>Day</th><th>Exercises</th><th>Duration</th><th>QR code</th></tr>
<tr>
<td rowspan="3">7</td>
<td>Wall Cross Body Crunches 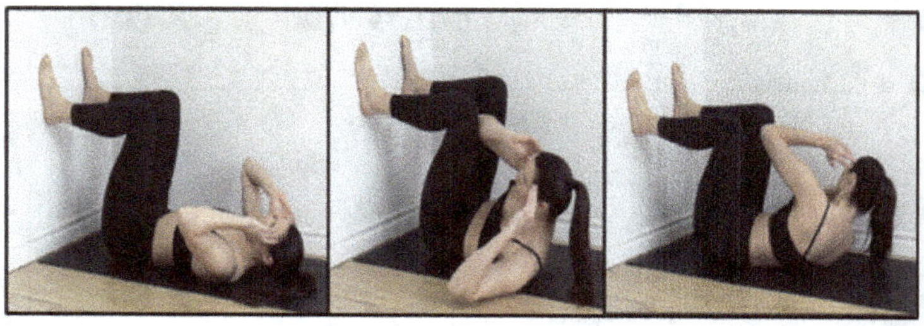</td>
<td>7 mins</td>
<td rowspan="3">https://youtu.be/GIvZXyfmCXU?si=1oUoewpytb3WWklq</td>
</tr>
<tr>
<td>Wall Pilates 100's 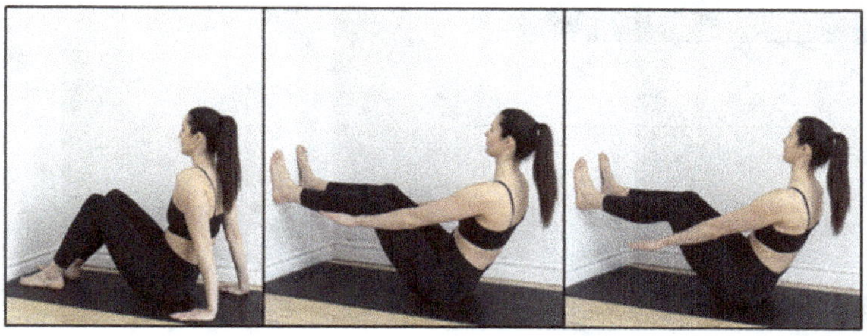</td>
<td>7 mins</td>
</tr>
<tr>
<td>Wall plank 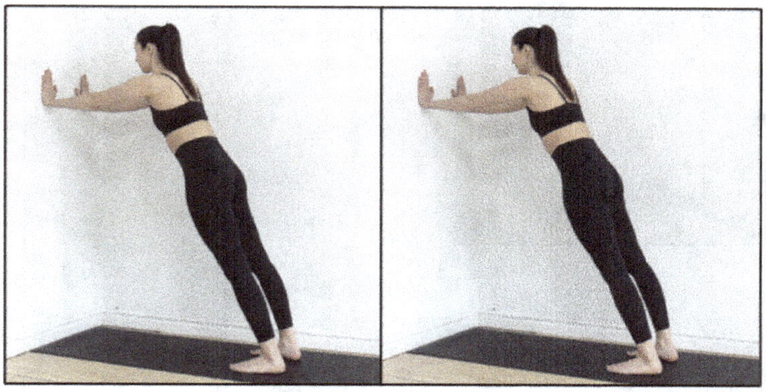</td>
<td>7 mins</td>
</tr>
</table>

WEEK 6 : Progressive Routines for Building Confidence 2/2

WEEK 6: PROGRESSIVE ROUTINE 1/2			
Day	Exercises	Duration	QR code
1	Wall Pilates 100's 	7 mins	https://youtu.be/vWBOW8b2JNo?si=z7GOeETehqRtdh6j
	Wall Shoulder Taps 	7 mins	
	Wall Push Ups 	7 mins	

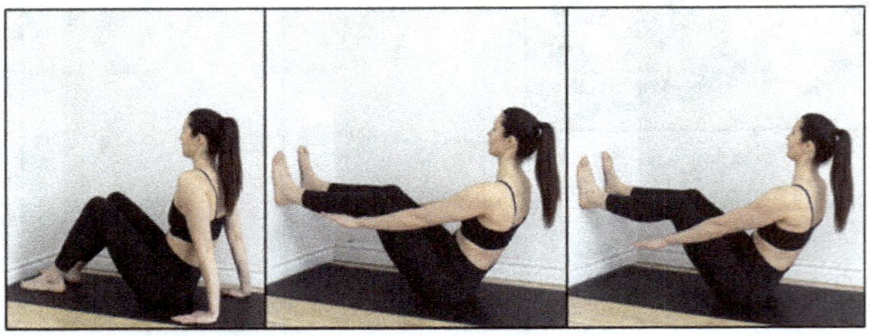

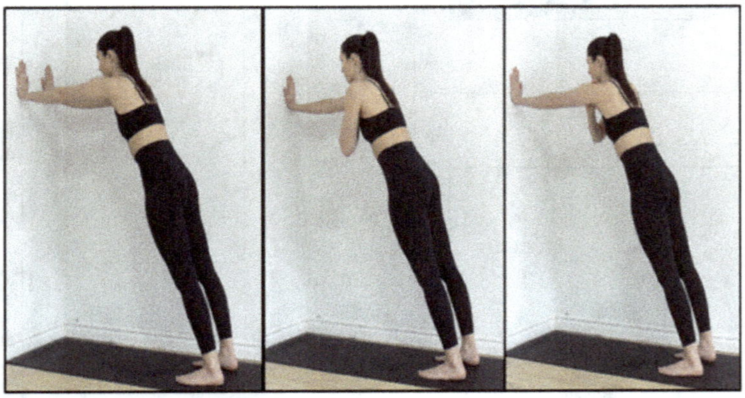

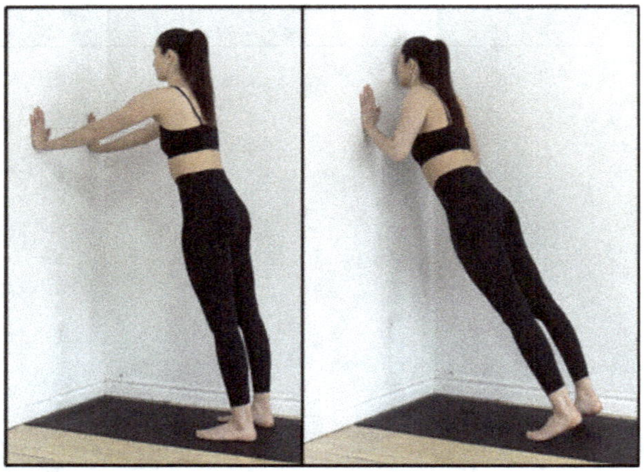

WEEK 6: PROGRESSIVE ROUTINE 1/2			
Da y	Exercises	Duration	QR code
2	Wall Squats Wall Side to Side Lunges	7 mins 7 mins	https://youtu .be/QHLdEi S- 1kk?si=scii9 - OelGanjyok

<table>
<tr><td colspan="4" align="center">WEEK 6: PROGRESSIVE ROUTINE 1/2</td></tr>
<tr><td>Day</td><td align="center">Exercises</td><td>Duration</td><td>QR code</td></tr>
<tr><td rowspan="2">3</td><td align="center">Wall Reverse Lunges 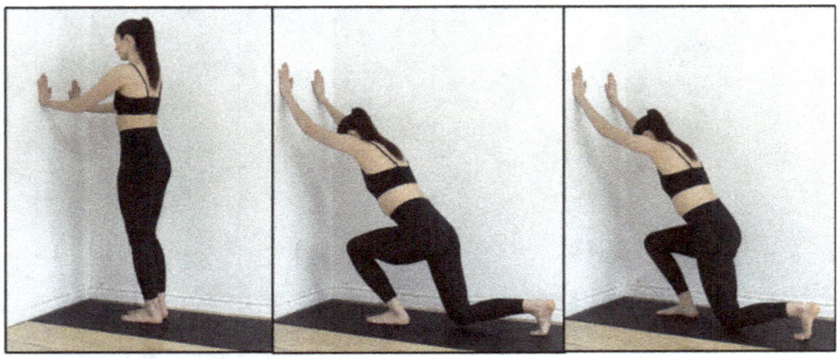</td><td></td><td rowspan="2">https://youtu.be/-qElRPYNuTg?si=fYSNmB6CWIIloB0q</td></tr>
<tr><td align="center">Wall Cross Body Crunches

Wall Pilates 100's 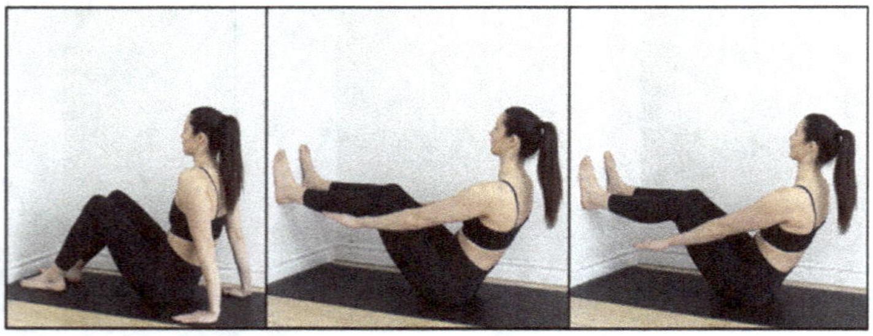

Wall plank</td><td>7 mins

7 mins

7 mins</td></tr>
</table>

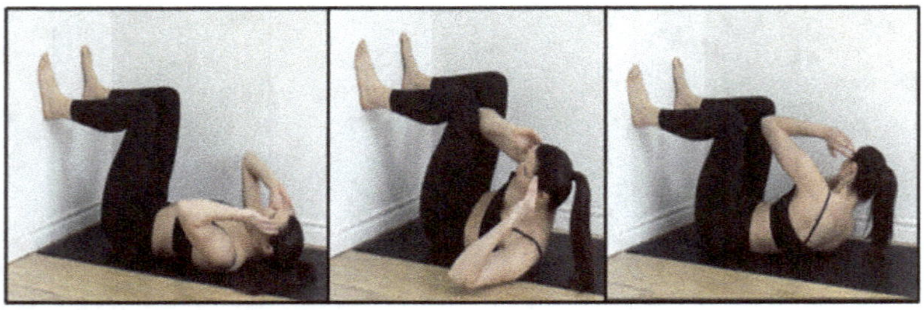

<table>
<tr><th colspan="4" align="center">WEEK 6: PROGRESSIVE ROUTINE 1/2</th></tr>
<tr><th>Day</th><th>Exercises</th><th>Duration</th><th>QR code</th></tr>
<tr>
<td rowspan="2">4</td>
<td>

Wall Push Ups 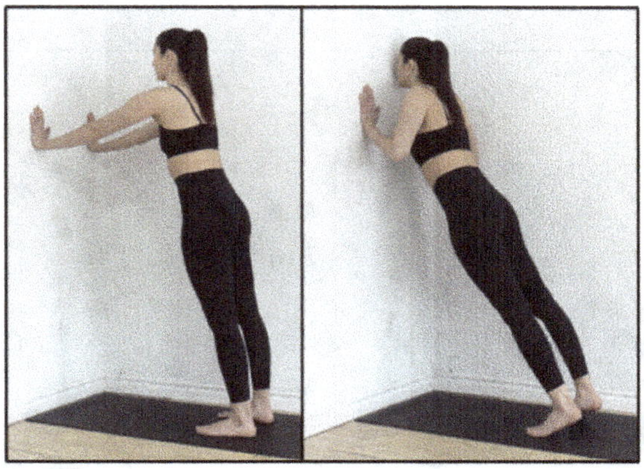

Wall Tricep Press

</td>
<td>7 mins

7 mins</td>
<td>

https://youtu.be/jQbmjHygJig?si=ObzjEjac6cW–MIOP

</td>
</tr>
</table>

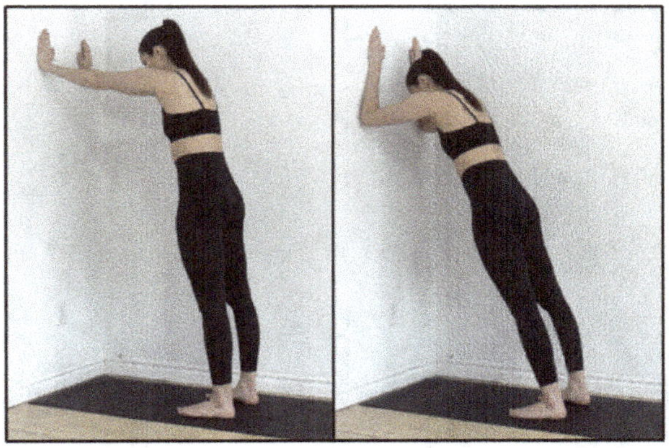

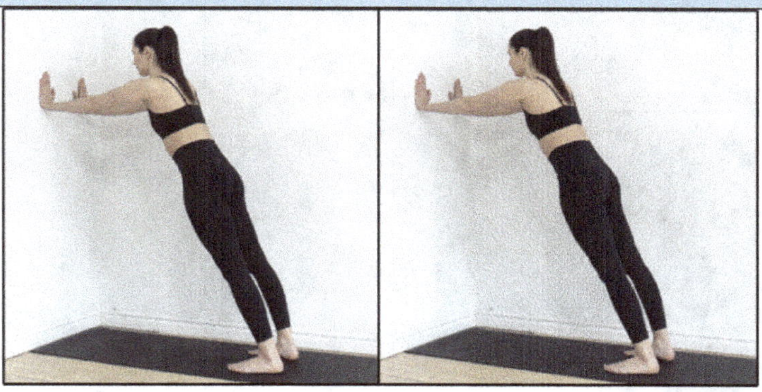

<table>
<tr><td colspan="4" align="center">WEEK 6: PROGRESSIVE ROUTINE 1/2</td></tr>
<tr><td>Day</td><td align="center">Exercises</td><td>Duration</td><td>QR code</td></tr>
<tr><td rowspan="3">5</td><td align="center">Wall Arm Angels</td><td>7 mins</td><td></td></tr>
<tr><td align="center">Wall Pilates 100's</td><td>7 mins</td><td rowspan="2">https://youtu.be/xXrdOQ-8qWE?si=0lQqgf_nFFRaysvx</td></tr>
<tr><td align="center">Wall Shoulder Taps</td><td>7 mins</td></tr>
</table>

<table>
<tr><th colspan="4" style="text-align:center">WEEK 6: PROGRESSIVE ROUTINE 1/2</th></tr>
<tr><th>Day</th><th style="text-align:center">Exercises</th><th>Duration</th><th>QR code</th></tr>
<tr>
<td rowspan="3">6</td>
<td>Wall Push Ups 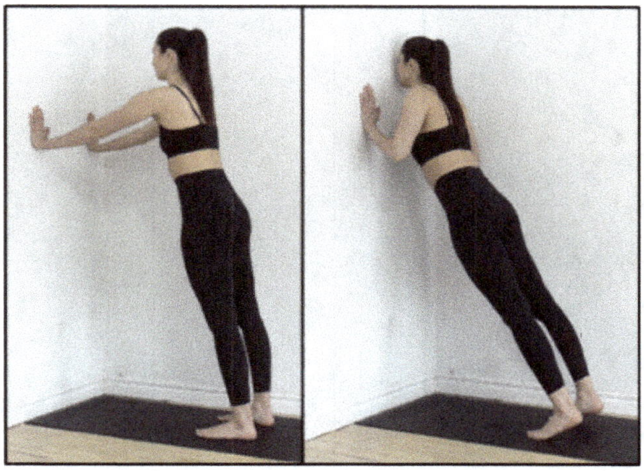</td>
<td>7 mins</td>
<td></td>
</tr>
<tr>
<td>Wall Squats 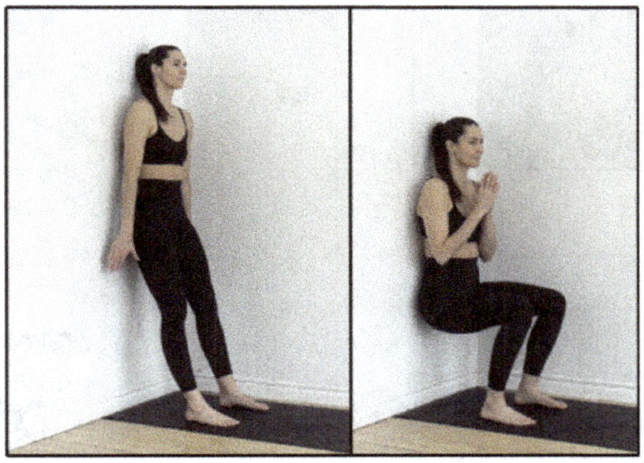</td>
<td>7 mins</td>
<td>https://youtu.be/b0W1cFbgITI?si=yRsXwr7DGZtt0ljf</td>
</tr>
<tr>
<td>Wall Side Lunges (Right) 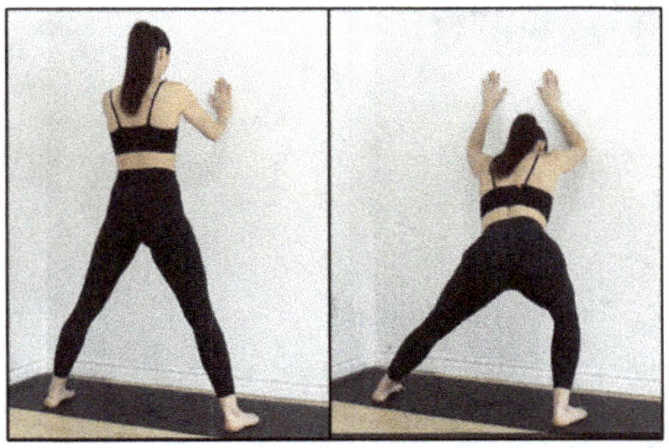</td>
<td>7 mins</td>
<td></td>
</tr>
</table>

<table>
<tr><th colspan="4">WEEK 6: PROGRESSIVE ROUTINE 1/2</th></tr>
<tr><th>Day</th><th>Exercises</th><th>Duration</th><th>QR code</th></tr>
<tr>
<td rowspan="2">7</td>
<td>Wall Side Lunges (Left)</td>
<td>7 mins</td>
<td></td>
</tr>
<tr>
<td>Wall Reach Through Crunches

Wall Pilates 100's

Wall plank</td>
<td>7 mins

7 mins</td>
<td>https://youtu.be/6PgW41Eluas?si=YoLAg_JoO48sZFA4</td>
</tr>
</table>

WEEK 6: PROGRESSIVE ROUTINE 1/2			
Day	Exercises	Duration	QR code
		7 mins	

	WEEK 7: OVERCOMING PLATEAUS AND CHALLENGES 1/2		
Day	**Exercises**	**Duration**	QR code
1	Wall Pilates 100's	7 mins	
	Wall Commando plank	7 mins	https://youtu.be/omrVb9gs37I?si=DbmdJgEfYUhy11eW
	Wall Push Ups	7 mins	

WEEK 7: OVERCOMING PLATEAUS AND CHALLENGES 1/2			
Day	Exercises	Duration	QR code
2	**Wall Squats** 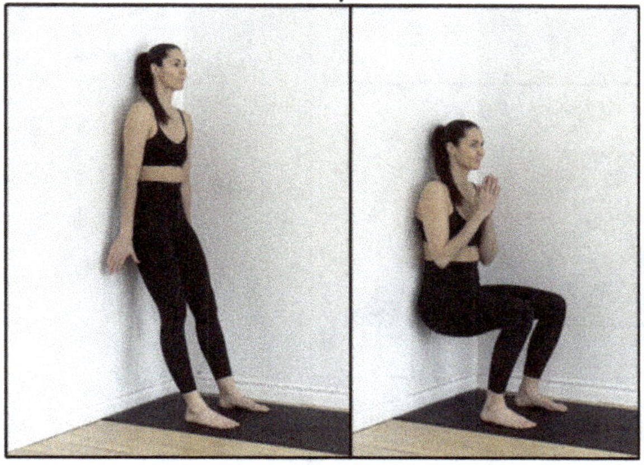	7 mins	
	Wall Side Lunges (Right) 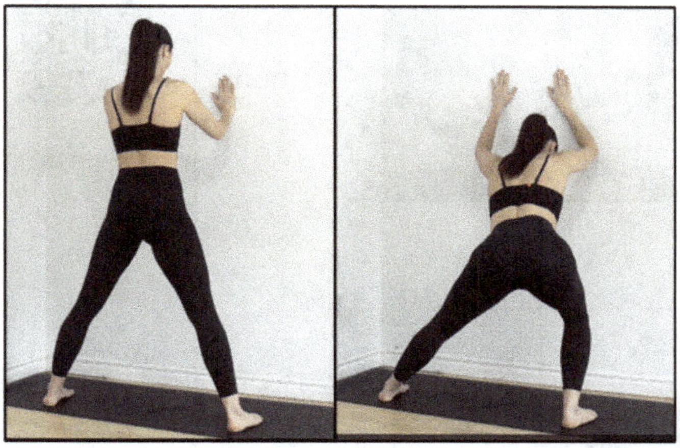	7 mins	https://youtu.be/ -8rAHM0TYDk?si= VhYGikfyQOM4U eYB
	Wall Side Lunges (Left) 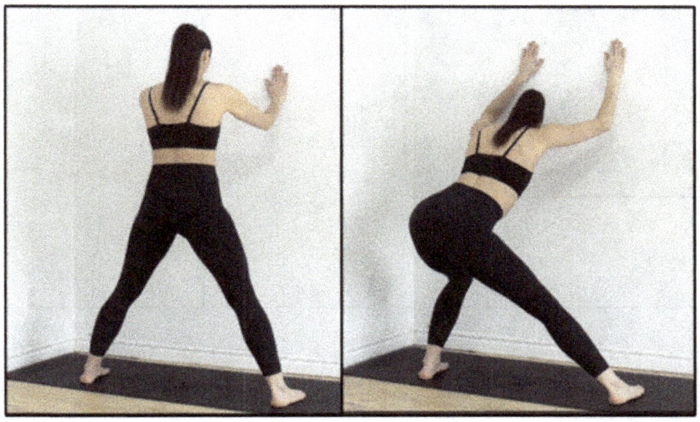	7 mins	

WEEK 7: OVERCOMING PLATEAUS AND CHALLENGES 1/2			
Day	Exercises	Duration	QR code
3	Wall Reach Through Crunches 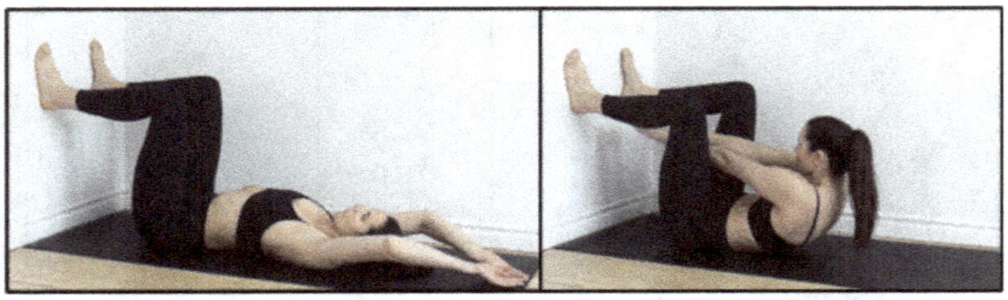	6 mins	
	Wall Pilates 100's 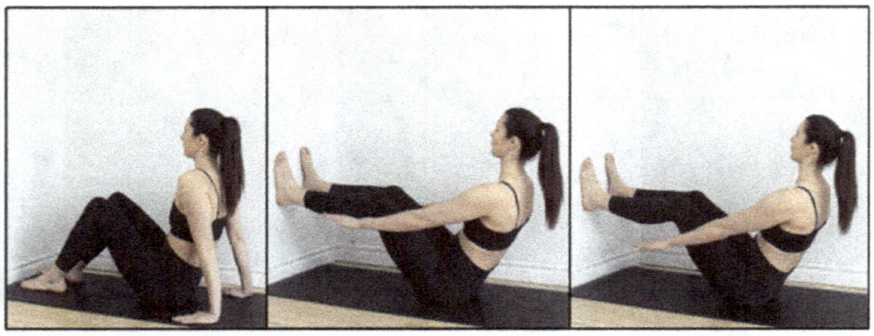	7 mins	https://youtu.be/2FRGWtUShro?si=h8_JOTawxDtkoR8l
	Wall plank 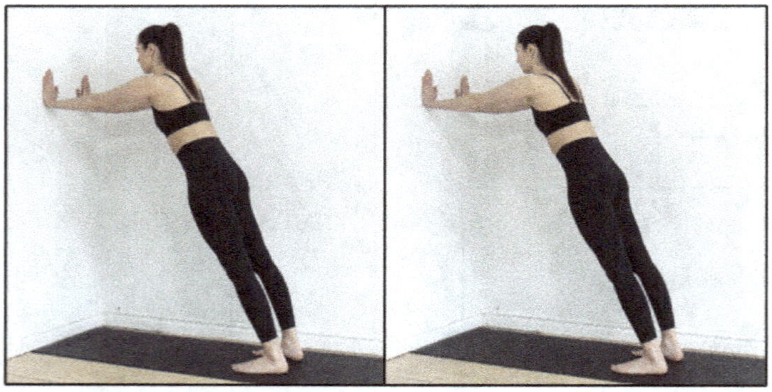	7 mins	

<table>
<tr><th colspan="4">WEEK 7: OVERCOMING PLATEAUS AND CHALLENGES 1/2</th></tr>
<tr><th>Day</th><th>Exercises</th><th>Duration</th><th>QR code</th></tr>
<tr><td rowspan="3">4</td><td>Wall Push Ups
 </td><td>7 mins</td><td rowspan="3">https://youtu.be/7wqt2JdqAH8?si=wwXlPvhCVu251pnL</td></tr>
<tr><td>Wall Tricep Press
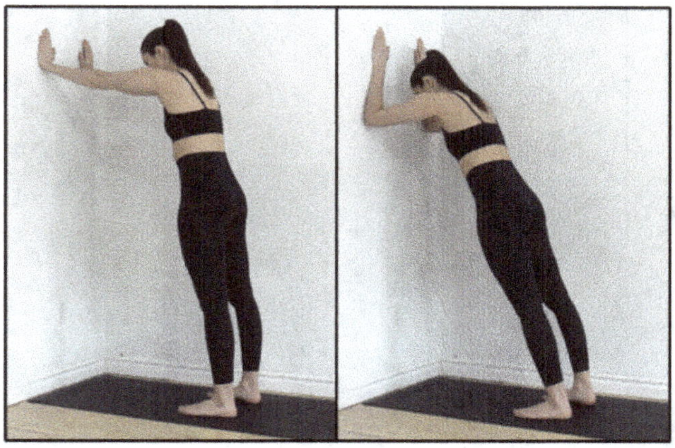</td><td>7 mins</td></tr>
<tr><td>Wall Arm Butterflies
 </td><td>7 mins</td></tr>
</table>

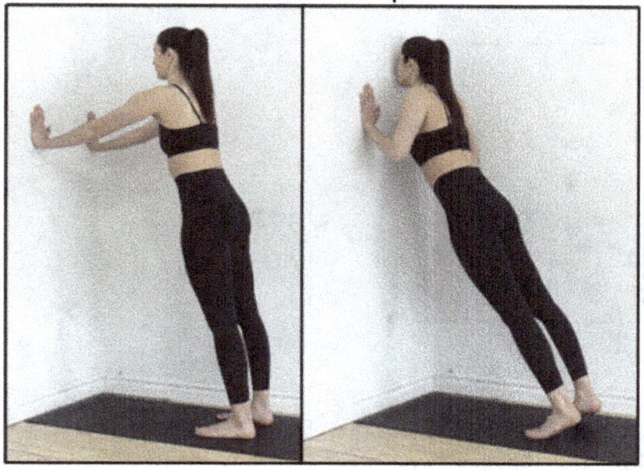

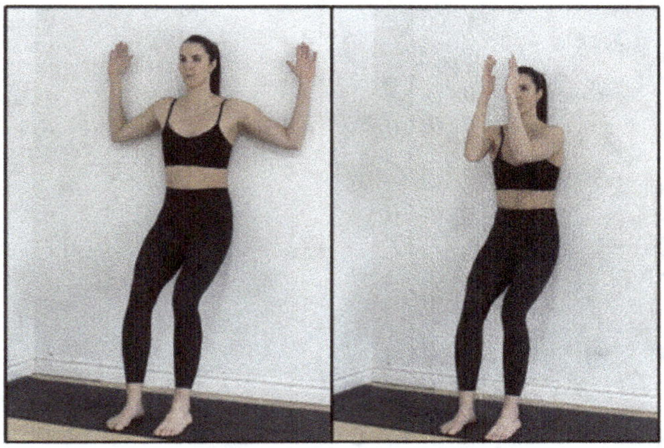

WEEK 7: OVERCOMING PLATEAUS AND CHALLENGES 1/2			
Day	**Exercises**	**Duration**	QR code
5	Wall Pilates 100's	7 mins	https://youtu.be/NjT5yTsUGJw?si=2GJmvNT56HrYiRk2
	Wall Shoulder Taps 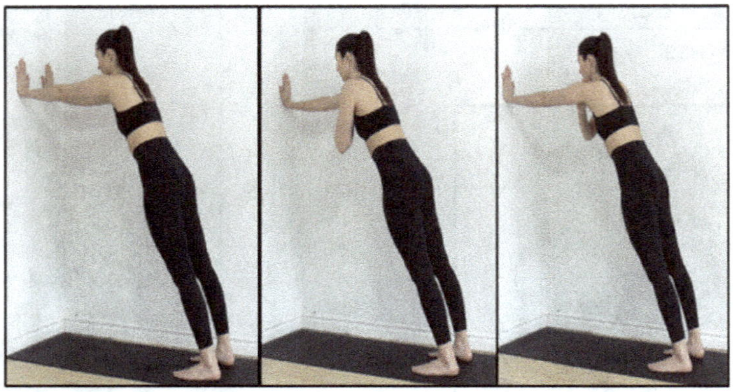	7 mins	
	Wall Push Ups	7 mins	

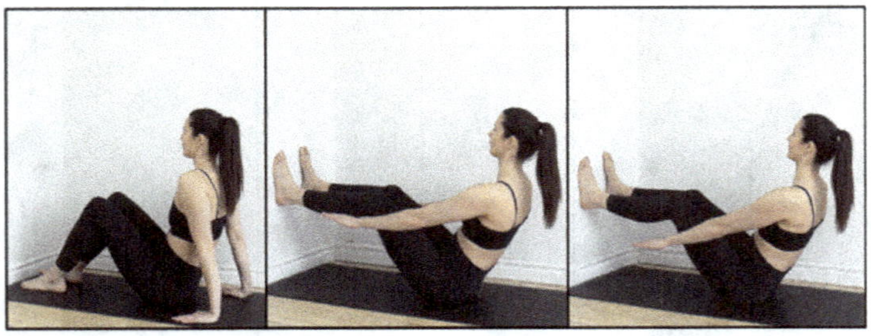

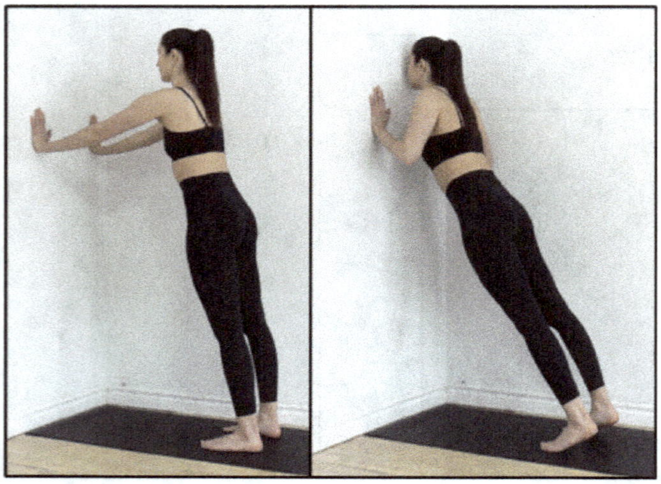

<table>
<tr><th colspan="4">WEEK 7: OVERCOMING PLATEAUS AND CHALLENGES 1/2</th></tr>
<tr><th>Day</th><th>Exercises</th><th>Duration</th><th>QR code</th></tr>
<tr><td rowspan="3">6</td><td>Wall Squats 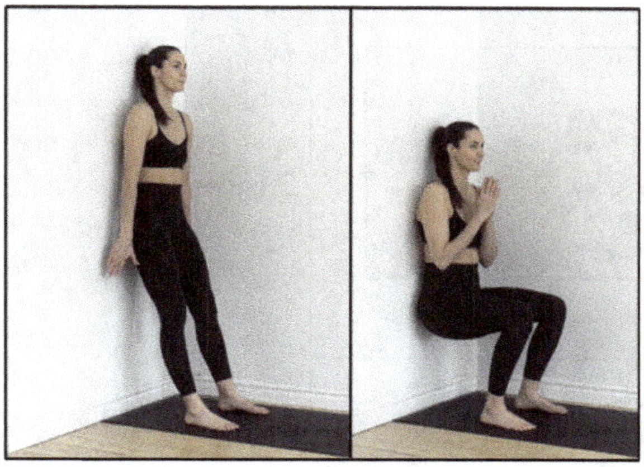</td><td>7 mins</td><td rowspan="3">https://youtu.be/9bMqLIu0zpo?si=nGSFrVgc0lis5HNk</td></tr>
<tr><td>Wall Side to Side Lunges 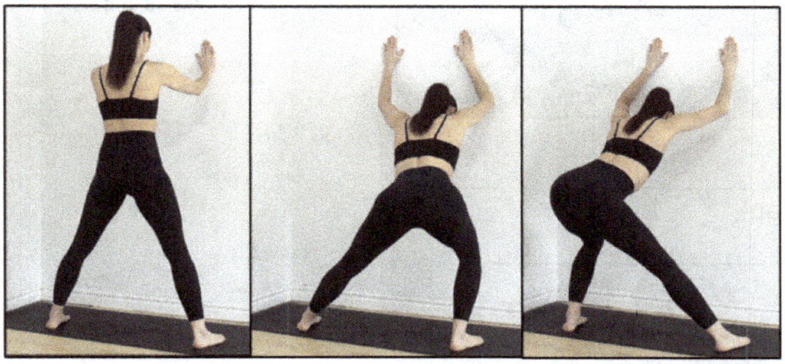</td><td>7 mins</td></tr>
<tr><td>Wall Reverse Lunges 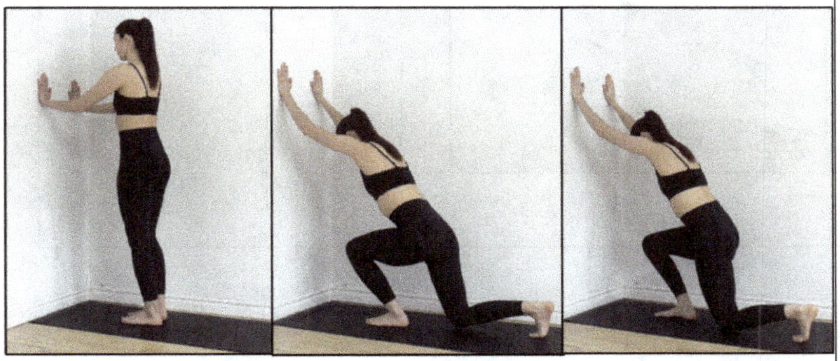</td><td>7 mins</td></tr>
</table>

<table>
<tr><th colspan="4">WEEK 7: OVERCOMING PLATEAUS AND CHALLENGES 1/2</th></tr>
<tr><th>Day</th><th>Exercises</th><th>Durati on</th><th>QR code</th></tr>
<tr>
<td rowspan="3">7</td>
<td>Wall Reach Through Crunches</td>
<td>7 mins</td>
<td rowspan="3">https://youtu.be/ 2mxjnyh6l70?si=F TMOFD60WZrcl3 Av</td>
</tr>
<tr>
<td>Wall Pilates 100's</td>
<td>7 mins</td>
</tr>
<tr>
<td>Wall plank</td>
<td>7 mins</td>
</tr>
</table>

WEEK 8: Overcoming Plateaus and Challenges 2/2

WEEK 8: OVERCOMING PLATEAUS AND CHALLENGES 2/2			
Day	Exercises	Duration	QR code
1	Wall Pilates 100's 	7 mins	https://youtu.be/7_Xggf3gm6c?si=mqnepG4I2tD3lES9
	Wall commando plank 	7 mins	
	Wall Push Ups 	7 mins	

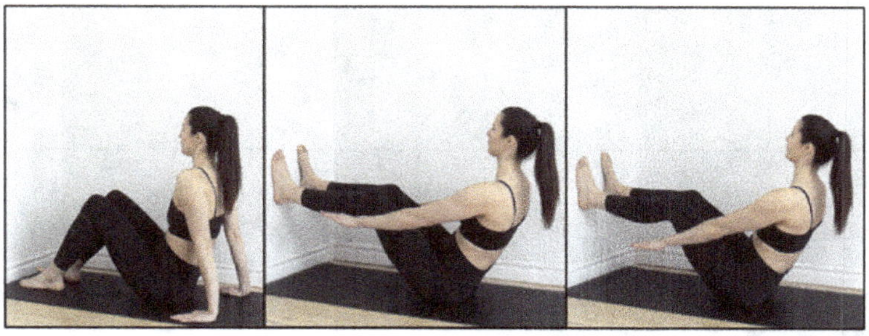

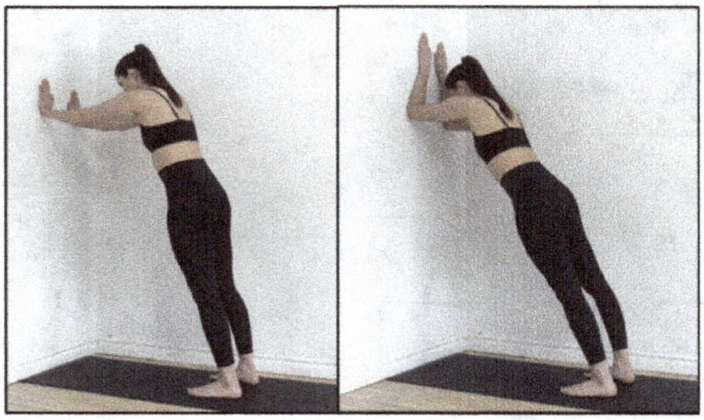

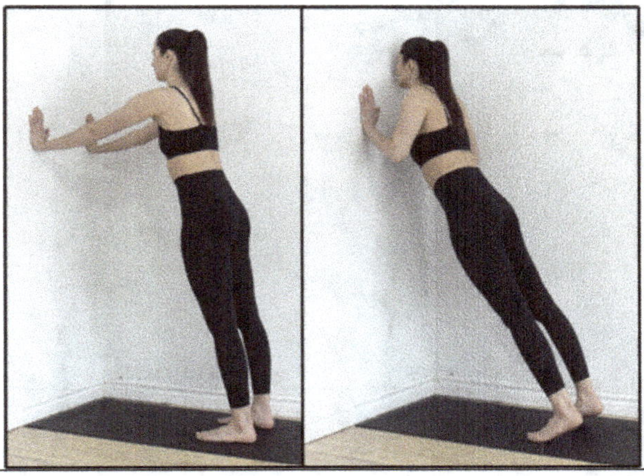

WEEK 8: OVERCOMING PLATEAUS AND CHALLENGES 2/2			
Day	Exercises	Duration	QR code
2	Wall Squats	7 mins	https://youtu.be/jXsXzO90Gtc?si=r_n16aLJlaORI9d1
	Wall Side to side lunges	7 mins	
	Wall reverse lunges	7 mins	

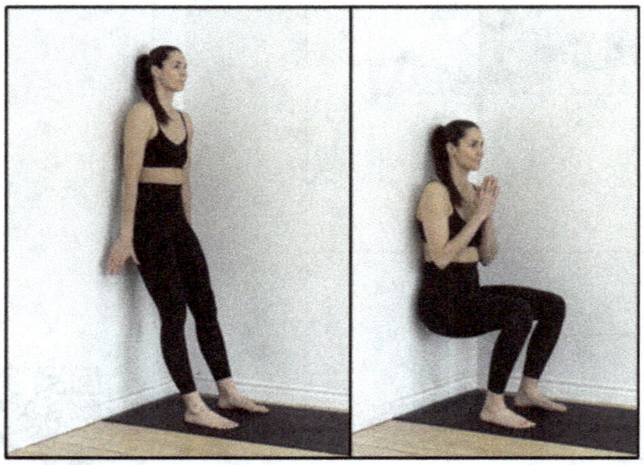

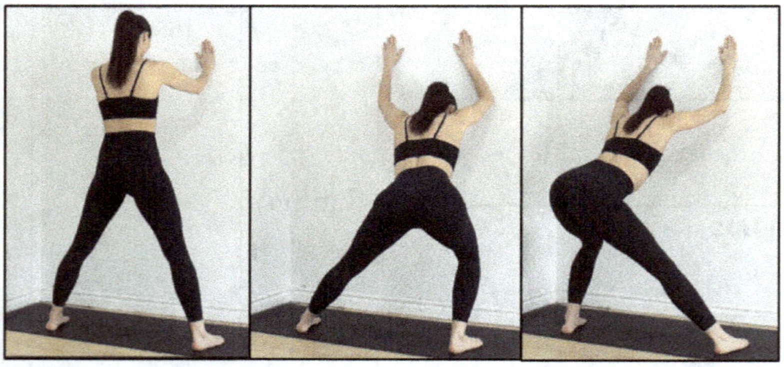

<table>
<tr><th colspan="4">WEEK 8: OVERCOMING PLATEAUS AND CHALLENGES 2/2</th></tr>
<tr><th>Day</th><th>Exercises</th><th>Duration</th><th>QR code</th></tr>
<tr>
<td rowspan="2">3</td>
<td>Wall Reach Through Crunches</td>
<td></td>
<td rowspan="2">https://youtu.be/JSmOvDhNf4A?si=_LpcCgoELPckTHpF</td>
</tr>
<tr>
<td>Wall Pilates 100's

Wall plank</td>
<td>7 mins

7 mins

7 mins</td>
</tr>
</table>

Day	Exercises	Duration	QR code
4	Wall Push Ups Wall Tricep Press	7 mins 7 mins	https://youtu.be/1NVtIIY0fnI?si=34rV7ph3aD2tYT40

<table>
<tr><th colspan="4">WEEK 8: OVERCOMING PLATEAUS AND CHALLENGES 2/2</th></tr>
<tr><th>Day</th><th>Exercises</th><th>Duration</th><th>QR code</th></tr>
<tr><td rowspan="3">5</td><td>Wall Arm Butterflies 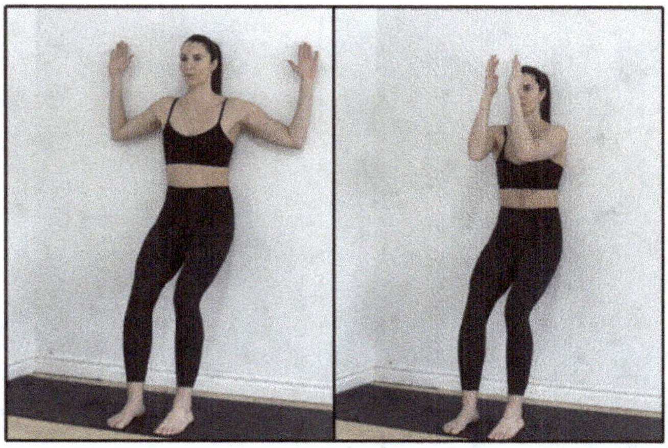</td><td>7 mins</td><td></td></tr>
<tr><td>Wall Pilates 100's 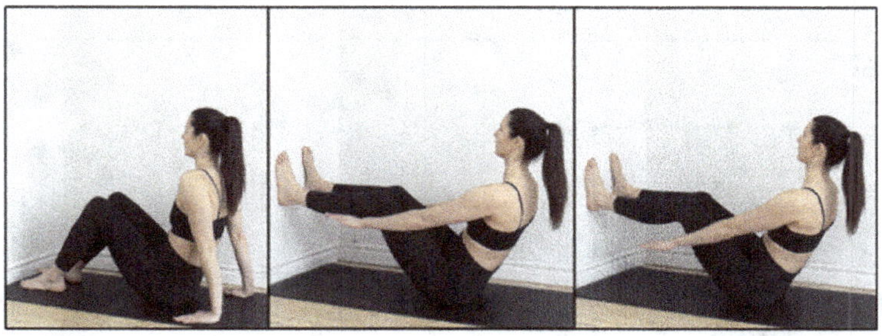</td><td>7 mins</td><td rowspan="2">https://youtu.be/QSTnpZBVa_8?si=tS1GoOtMSvKVON_J</td></tr>
<tr><td>Wall commando plank 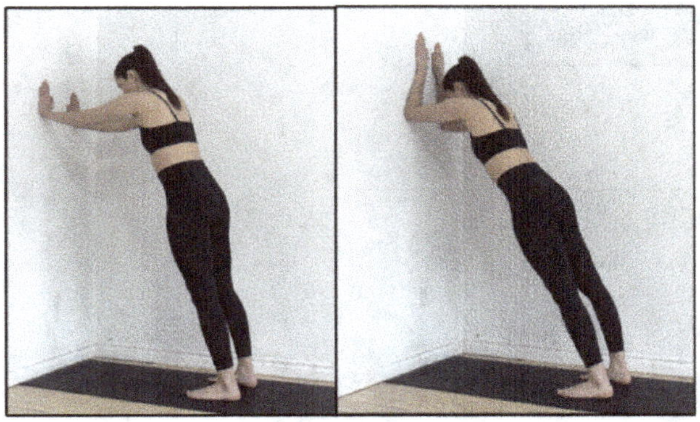</td><td>7 mins</td></tr>
</table>

<table>
<tr><th colspan="4">WEEK 8: OVERCOMING PLATEAUS AND CHALLENGES 2/2</th></tr>
<tr><th>Day</th><th>Exercises</th><th>Duration</th><th>QR code</th></tr>
<tr><td rowspan="3">6</td><td>Wall Push Ups</td><td>7 mins</td><td></td></tr>
<tr><td>Wall Squat</td><td>7 mins</td><td>https://youtu.be/E4J_7rkp7w8?si=r4w7oKPe_PIYBFPR</td></tr>
<tr><td>Wall Side to side Lunges</td><td>7 mins</td><td></td></tr>
</table>

<table>
<tr><th colspan="4">WEEK 8: OVERCOMING PLATEAUS AND CHALLENGES 2/2</th></tr>
<tr><th>Day</th><th>Exercises</th><th>Duration</th><th>QR code</th></tr>
<tr><td rowspan="4">7</td><td>Wall reverse lunges</td><td>7 mins</td><td rowspan="4">https://youtu.be/MQuTrOeEEvo?si=adDqXRH4jv-YC3mU</td></tr>
<tr><td>Wall Reach Through Crunches</td><td></td></tr>
<tr><td>Wall Pilates 100's</td><td>7 mins</td></tr>
<tr><td></td><td>7 mins</td></tr>
</table>

<table>
<tr><td colspan="4" align="center">WEEK 8: OVERCOMING PLATEAUS AND CHALLENGES 2/2</td></tr>
<tr><td>Day</td><td align="center">Exercises</td><td>Duration</td><td>QR code</td></tr>
<tr><td></td><td align="center"></td><td>7 mins</td><td></td></tr>
<tr><td></td><td align="center">Wall plank 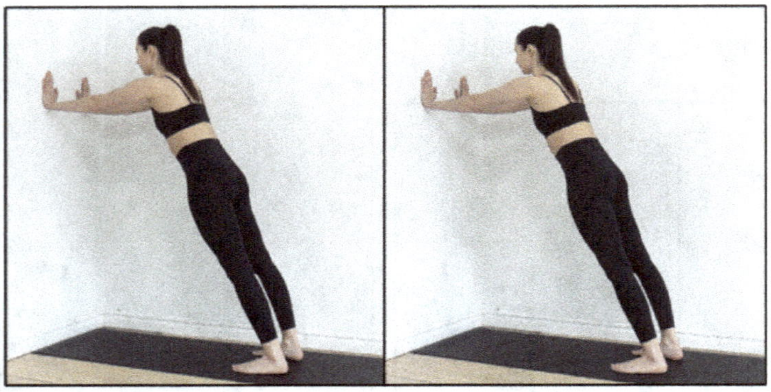</td><td></td><td></td></tr>
</table>

Chapter 7: Wall Pilates for Special Circumstances - Pregnancy

Pregnancy, a miraculous and transformative journey, introduces unique physical and emotional changes in a woman's life. As the body adapts to accommodate new life, it becomes essential to approach fitness with a mindful and tailored perspective. In this section, we delve into the intricacies of Safe Wall Pilates Practices for Expectant Mothers, providing detailed insights into the importance of these practices for the well-being of both the mother and the growing baby.

Pregnancy brings forth a series of physiological changes that influence the musculoskeletal system, balance, and overall comfort. These changes may manifest as back pain, muscle weakness, and alterations in posture, creating the need for a specialized approach to exercise. Wall Pilates, with its emphasis on controlled movements and gentle support, emerges as an ideal fitness modality to address these challenges. By providing a nurturing environment, Wall Pilates becomes a trusted companion throughout the various stages of pregnancy.

Mindful Modifications for a Supportive Practice

As pregnancy progresses, modifications in traditional Pilates exercises become imperative to ensure the safety of both the mother and the baby. Wall Pilates, with its supportive structure, facilitates mindful adaptations. For example, abdominal exercises can be modified to emphasize pelvic floor engagement, fostering core strength without placing undue stress on the changing anatomy. The approach centers around creating a safe and supportive space for expectant mothers to maintain their fitness journey.

Emphasizing Pelvic Floor Engagement

A cornerstone of safe Wall Pilates practices for expectant mothers involves placing a deliberate focus on pelvic floor engagement. Strengthening these muscles not only supports the pelvic region but also contributes to improved posture and stability. Exercises such as wall-supported squats, gentle leg lifts, and pelvic tilts become integral components of the routine, promoting a healthy pelvic floor function during and after pregnancy.

Addressing Common Concerns

Throughout pregnancy, women may encounter concerns related to balance, joint discomfort, and overall fatigue. Safe Wall Pilates practices take these concerns into account by offering exercises that enhance balance through the reliable support of the wall. These exercises also aim to alleviate joint stress and provide a gentle energy boost, addressing the unique needs and challenges associated with each trimester.

Breathing Techniques for Relaxation

Creating a calming and relaxing environment is paramount for expectant mothers, and incorporating mindful breathing techniques achieves just that. Safe Wall Pilates practices integrate diaphragmatic breathing, encouraging a rhythmic breath-to-movement connection. These techniques not only enhance relaxation but also contribute to improved oxygen flow, benefiting both the mother and the baby. The focus remains on cultivating a positive connection between the mother and her changing body through intentional breathwork.

Hydration and Nutrition Tips

Staying adequately hydrated and maintaining a balanced nutritional intake are critical aspects of a healthy pregnancy. Safe Wall Pilates practices incorporate practical tips on hydration and nutrition, emphasizing the importance of nourishing the body to support the increased demands of both pregnancy and exercise. These guidelines empower expectant mothers to make informed choices that contribute to their overall well-being.

Consultation with Health Professionals

Before embarking on any exercise routine during pregnancy, seeking guidance from healthcare professionals is paramount. Safe Wall Pilates practices underscore the importance of consulting with obstetricians or midwives to ensure that the chosen exercises align with individual health conditions and the specific needs of the pregnancy. This collaborative approach ensures a safe and tailored fitness journey for expectant mothers.

Empowering Maternal Well-being:

Incorporating safe Wall Pilates practices into the journey of pregnancy is an important suggestion. It encourages expectant mothers to celebrate their bodies, stay connected with their changing selves, and embrace the holistic benefits that Wall Pilates can bring to maternal well-being. The overarching message is one of empowerment and self-care, emphasizing the transformative and positive impact that a mindful Pilates practice can have on the holistic health of expectant mothers. Safe Wall Pilates Practices for Expectant Mothers stands as a comprehensive guide, fostering a sense of confidence and empowerment for women during this beautiful and transformative phase of life.

Trimester 1: Nurturing a Foundation of Strength

The first trimester is a crucial period marked by the initial adaptations in the body to accommodate the growing fetus. Adapting Wall Pilates routines during this stage involves laying a foundation of strength while respecting the body's evolving needs. Gentle exercises that focus on core stability, pelvic floor engagement, and controlled breathing become integral components. Wall-supported squats, modified plank positions, and pelvic tilts offer a balanced approach to building strength without overwhelming the body.

Wall Plank with Pelvic Floor Emphasis: Begin in a plank position with feet against the wall, emphasizing pelvic floor engagement. Hold for 20 seconds, gradually increasing duration.

Wall Squats for Lower Body Strength: Perform squats with the back against the wall to activate lower body muscles. Aim for 3 sets of 15, maintaining proper form.

Gentle Leg Lifts: While lying on the back, lift legs against the wall to target the lower abdominal region. Focus on controlled movements and engage the lower abs.

These exercises provide a gentle introduction to Wall Pilates, fostering strength and stability in preparation for the subsequent stages of pregnancy.

Trimester 2: Embracing Fluidity and Comfort

As the body adapts to the changing weight distribution and hormonal fluctuations, the second trimester offers an opportunity to embrace fluid and comfortable movements. Wall Pilates routines can be adapted to include exercises that enhance flexibility, promote relaxation, and alleviate potential discomfort. Incorporating gentle stretches, breathing techniques, and exercises that cater to the changing center of gravity become key elements during this stage.

Wall Chest Opener: Stretch chest muscles by placing hands on the wall and gently leaning forward. Breathe deeply, feeling the stretch across the chest.

Wall Hamstring Stretch: Hinge at the hips with one foot on the wall for a hamstring stretch. Focus on controlled movements and feel the stretch in the back of the leg.

Wall Roll-Downs for Spinal Articulation: Slowly articulate the spine down the wall, engaging core muscles. Aim for 3 sets of 12, moving one vertebra at a time.

These adapted routines foster a sense of fluidity, enhancing comfort and relaxation for expectant mothers during the second trimester.

Trimester 3: Prioritizing Comfort and Preparation

The third trimester brings the anticipation of the upcoming childbirth, requiring a focus on comfort and preparation. Adapting Wall Pilates routines during this stage involves choosing exercises that prioritize comfort, promote optimal fetal positioning, and prepare the body for labor. Emphasis is placed on controlled movements that avoid strain, with a focus on breathing techniques that can be beneficial during delivery.

Wall Supported Breathing Techniques: Utilize the wall for support while practicing diaphragmatic breathing. Emphasize relaxation and rhythmic breath-to-movement connection.

Gentle Wall Pilates Roll-Up: Combine a traditional roll-up with wall support, articulating the spine with control. Foster a sense of relaxation and mindfulness.

Wall Side Plank for Oblique Engagement: Engage obliques with a side plank against the wall. Lift hips high, maintaining a straight line from head to heels.

These adapted routines in the third trimester prioritize comfort, relaxation, and preparation for the upcoming birthing experience.

Guiding Principles for Adapting Wall Pilates

Listen to Your Body: Each woman's pregnancy journey is unique. Pay attention to your body's signals and modify exercises accordingly.

Consultation with Health Professionals: Before embarking on any exercise routine during pregnancy, consult with obstetricians or midwives to ensure alignment with individual health conditions.

Mindful Breathing: Integrate diaphragmatic breathing throughout each routine to enhance relaxation and oxygen flow.

Supportive Wall: Utilize the wall for support in various exercises, ensuring stability and a sense of security.

Empowering Women Through Adaptable Wall Pilates: Adapting Wall Pilates routines for different pregnancy stages is an empowering and holistic approach to maternal fitness. By tailoring exercises to align with the unique needs of each trimester, expectant mothers can embrace the transformative journey with confidence and well-being. This chapter serves as a comprehensive guide, providing not only a repertoire of adapted exercises but also a philosophy that honors the beauty and strength inherent in every stage of pregnancy. Through adaptable Wall Pilates practices, women can nurture their physical and emotional well-being, fostering a connection with their changing bodies and the new life they are bringing into the world.

Trimester	Exercise	Description	Benefit	Risk/Suggestion
1st	Pelvic Tilts	Lie on your back with knees bent. Tilt pelvis backward, then forward, engaging core muscles. Repeat for 10-15 reps.	Strengthens pelvic floor muscles, improves posture, and reduces lower back discomfort.	Avoid lying flat on back after the first trimester. If uncomfortable, perform while lying on your side.
	Modified Push-Ups	Perform against a wall or countertop, keeping body aligned and elbows close to the body. Aim for 10-15 reps.	Strengthens upper body muscles without straining the abdomen.	Avoid full push-ups, especially as pregnancy progresses. Keep hips aligned with shoulders to avoid strain on the lower back.
	Seated Leg Lifts	Sit on a chair with feet flat on the floor. Raise one leg at a time, extending it straight out in front of you, then lower it back down to the starting position. Alternate between legs for the desired number of repetitions..	Strengthens and tones leg muscles.	Keep spine straight and avoid leaning back excessively.
	Wall Squats	Stand with back against a wall, feet hip-width apart. Slide down into a squat position, then push back up. Do 10-15 reps.	Strengthens quadriceps, hamstrings, and glutes. Improves lower body strength and endurance.	Avoid squatting too low to prevent strain on the knees. Keep knees aligned with toes.

Trimester	Exercise	Description	Benefit	Risk/Suggestion
	Wall Push-Ups	Stand arm's length from a wall, lean forward, and place palms flat against the wall. Perform push-ups by bending elbows and pushing back. Aim for 10-15 reps.	Strengthens chest, arms, and shoulders.	Maintain a straight line from head to heels to avoid strain on the lower back.
	Kegel Exercises	Sit or lie down comfortably. Tighten pelvic floor muscles as if stopping the flow of urine. Hold for a few seconds, then release. Repeat 10-15 times.	Strengthens pelvic floor muscles, aids in bladder control, and prepares for childbirth.	Avoid overexertion or holding breath while performing Kegel exercises.
	Standing Side Leg Raises	Stand next to a wall or chair for support. Lift one leg out to the side, then lower it back down. Do 10 reps on each side.	Strengthens hip abductor muscles and improves balance.	Hold onto a stable surface for balance if needed. Avoid leaning excessively to one side.
	Modified Plank	Kneel on all fours, extend one leg back at a time, keeping hips level. Hold for 10-15 seconds, then switch legs.	Strengthens core muscles, including abdominals and lower back.	Avoid overarching the lower back or holding the position for too long. Listen to your body and rest as needed.
	Cat-Cow Stretch	Start on all fours, arch your back up like a cat, then release into a gentle sway like a cow. Repeat for 10-15 reps.	Improves flexibility and mobility in the spine.	Move slowly and gently, avoiding any sudden or jerky movements.
	Leg Circles	Lie on your side with legs extended, lift top leg and make small circles in the air. Repeat for 10 reps in each direction, then switch sides.	Strengthens hip muscles and improves hip mobility.	Keep movements controlled and within a comfortable range of motion. Avoid overarching the lower back or rotating hips excessively.

Trimester	Exercise	Description	Benefit	Risk/Suggestion
2nd	Wall Sit with Leg Lifts	Sit against a wall with knees bent at a 90-degree angle. Lift one leg straight out in front, then lower it back down. Alternate legs for 10 reps each.	Strengthens quadriceps, glutes, and hip flexors. Improves balance and stability.	Avoid holding the position for too long to prevent strain on the knees. Listen to your body and rest as needed.
	Seated Ball Squeeze	Sit on a chair with a small exercise ball between knees. Squeeze the ball gently, then release. Repeat for 10-15 reps.	Strengthens inner thigh muscles and pelvic floor. Improves pelvic stability and circulation.	Use a ball of appropriate size and firmness. Avoid excessive squeezing or holding breath.
	Modified Bridge	Lie on your back with knees bent and feet flat on the floor. Lift hips off the ground, squeezing glutes, then lower back down. Repeat for 10-15 reps.	Strengthens glutes, hamstrings, and lower back muscles. Improves core stability.	Avoid lying flat on back after the first trimester. If uncomfortable, perform while lying on your side. Engage pelvic floor muscles and avoid overarching the lower back.
	Side-Lying Leg Press	Lie on your side with bottom leg bent for support and top leg straight. Press top leg forward, then return to starting position. Do 10-15 reps on each side.	Strengthens outer thigh muscles and improves hip mobility.	Keep movements controlled and within a comfortable range of motion. Avoid rolling backward or forward.
	Wall Chest Stretch	Stand facing a wall with one hand against it at shoulder height. Rotate body away from the wall to feel a stretch in the chest. Hold for 15-30 seconds, then switch sides.	Relieves tension in chest muscles and opens up the shoulders.	Avoid overstretching or bouncing. Move gently into the stretch and hold at a comfortable range of motion.
	Deep Breathing Exercises	Sit or lie down comfortably. Take a deep breath in through your nose, allowing your belly to expand fully. Then, exhale slowly through your mouth, emptying your lungs completely. Repeat this breathing pattern throughout the exercise to promote relaxation and enhance your mind-body	Promotes relaxation, reduces stress, and increases oxygen flow to the baby.	Avoid holding breath or hyperventilating. Breathe naturally and rhythmically.

Trimester	Exercise	Description	Benefit	Risk/Suggestion
		connection. Repeat for 5-10 breaths.		
	Standing Side Leg Raises	Stand with one hand on a stable surface for support. Lift one leg out to the side, then lower it back down. Do 10 reps on each side.	Strengthens hip abductor muscles and improves balance.	Hold onto a stable surface for balance if needed. Avoid leaning excessively to one side.
	Arm Circles	Stand with arms extended to the sides. Make small circles with arms, gradually increasing the size. Repeat for 10-15 reps in each direction.	Improves shoulder mobility and strengthens shoulder muscles.	Keep movements controlled and within a comfortable range of motion. Avoid shrugging shoulders or tensing neck muscles.
	Pelvic Clocks	Lie on your back with knees bent and feet flat on the floor. Gently rock pelvis forward, backward, and side to side, following a clock-like pattern. Perform for 10-15 reps.	Enhances pelvic mobility, strengthens core muscles, and relieves lower back tension.	Perform movements slowly and mindfully. Avoid overarching the lower back or pressing down too hard.
	Modified Squats	Stand with feet hip-width apart, toes pointed slightly outward. Lower your body into a squat position, ensuring that your knees stay aligned with your toes. Once in the squat position, push through your heels to return to a standing position. Repeat this movement for the desired number of repetitions. Do 10-15 reps.	Strengthens quadriceps, hamstrings, and glutes. Improves lower body strength and endurance.	Avoid squatting too low to prevent strain on the knees. Keep knees aligned with toes.

Trimester	Exercise	Description	Benefit	Risk/Suggestion
3rd	Pelvic Tilts	Lie on your back with knees bent. Tilt pelvis backward, then forward, engaging core muscles. Repeat for 10-15 reps.	Strengthens pelvic floor muscles, improves posture, and reduces lower back discomfort.	Avoid lying flat on back after the first trimester. If uncomfortable, perform while lying on your side.
	Modified Push-Ups	Perform against a wall or countertop, keeping body aligned and elbows close	Strengthens upper body muscles without straining	Avoid full push-ups, especially as pregnancy progresses. Keep hips

	to the body. Aim for 10-15 reps.	the abdomen.	aligned with shoulders to avoid strain on the lower back.
Seated Leg Lifts	Sit on a chair with feet flat on the floor. Raise one leg at a time, extending it straight out in front of you, then lower it back down to the starting position. Alternate between legs for the desired number of repetitions.	Strengthens and tones leg muscles.	Keep spine straight and avoid leaning back excessively.
Wall Squats	Stand with back against a wall, feet hip-width apart. Slide down into a squat position, then push back up. Do 10-15 reps.	Strengthens quadriceps, hamstrings, and glutes. Improves lower body strength and endurance.	Avoid squatting too low to prevent strain on the knees. Keep knees aligned with toes.
Wall Push-Ups	Stand arm's length from a wall, lean forward, and place palms flat against the wall. Perform push-ups by bending elbows and pushing back. Aim for 10-15 reps.	Strengthens chest, arms, and shoulders.	Maintain a straight line from head to heels to avoid strain on the lower back.
Kegel Exercises	Sit or lie down comfortably. Tighten pelvic floor muscles as if stopping the flow of urine. Hold for a few seconds, then release. Repeat 10-15 times.	Strengthens pelvic floor muscles, aids in bladder control, and prepares for childbirth.	Avoid overexertion or holding breath while performing Kegel exercises.
Standing Side Leg Lifts	Stand next to a wall or chair for support. Lift one leg out to the side, then lower it back down. Do 10 reps on each side.	Strengthens hip abductor muscles and improves balance.	Hold onto a stable surface for balance if needed. Avoid leaning excessively to one side.
Modified Plank	Kneel on all fours, extend one leg back at a time, keeping hips level. Hold for 10-15 seconds, then switch legs.	Strengthens core muscles, including abdominals and lower back.	Avoid overarching the lower back or holding the position for too long. Listen to your body and rest as needed.
Cat-Cow Stretch	Start on all fours, arch your back up like a cat, then release into a gentle sway	Improves flexibility and mobility in the spine.	Move slowly and gently, avoiding any sudden or jerky movements.

		like a cow. Repeat for 10-15 reps.		
	Leg Circles	Lie on your side with legs extended, lift top leg and make small circles in the air. Repeat for 10 reps in each direction, then switch sides.	Strengthens hip muscles and improves hip mobility.	Keep movements controlled and within a comfortable range of motion. Avoid overarching the lower back or rotating hips excessively.

These exercises are designed to help pregnant women maintain fitness, strengthen muscles, and alleviate discomfort throughout each trimester of pregnancy. Always consult with a healthcare provider before starting any exercise program during pregnancy and listen to your body's cues to ensure safety and well-being.

Chapter 8: Wall Pilates for Special Circumstances- Your Period

Understanding Menstrual Changes and Exercise

In this comprehensive exploration, we delve into the intricate interplay between menstrual changes and exercise. Understanding the menstrual cycle is key to optimizing your Pilates practice, as it allows you to sync your workouts with your body's natural rhythms. We break down the four phases of the menstrual cycle—menstruation, the follicular phase, ovulation, and the luteal phase—and examine how hormonal fluctuations during each phase can impact energy levels, mood, and physical performance. By gaining insight into these changes, you can tailor your Pilates routine to align with your body's needs, optimizing both physical and mental well-being.

Menstrual cycles are a natural and integral part of a woman's reproductive health, accompanied by a series of physiological changes influenced by hormonal fluctuations. The menstrual cycle typically consists of four phases: menstrual, follicular, ovulatory, and luteal. Each phase brings its own set of hormonal variations, affecting energy levels, mood, and physical well-being.

Menstrual Phase (Days 1-5): This phase marks the onset of menstruation, characterized by the shedding of the uterine lining. Estrogen and progesterone levels are at their lowest. Many women experience fatigue and discomfort during this phase. Understanding these hormonal dynamics is crucial for adapting Wall Pilates routines.

Follicular Phase (Days 6-14): As estrogen levels gradually rise, you may experience increased energy levels and an uplifted mood. Women may find this phase more conducive to engaging in regular Wall Pilates workouts with moderate to high intensity. This phase is optimal for building strength and endurance.

Ovulatory Phase (Days 15-17): Ovulation occurs, and estrogen levels peak. Women might experience heightened energy, making it an excellent time for more intense Wall Pilates sessions. However, individual variations exist, and some may still prefer moderate workouts.

Luteal Phase (Days 18-28): Progesterone rises, potentially leading to increased body temperature and a sense of relaxation. This phase may be suitable for moderate-intensity Wall Pilates, with a focus on flexibility and mindful movements. However, discomfort and fatigue can vary among individuals.

Understanding these menstrual phases empowers women to align their Wall Pilates practice with their body's natural rhythm, optimizing the benefits of each workout while respecting the changing needs during different stages of the menstrual cycle. This knowledge encourages a compassionate and personalized approach to exercise, promoting overall well-being.

Listening to Your Body

Modifying Intensity and Duration: This section emphasizes the importance of attuning to your body's signals and adapting your Pilates practice accordingly. We recognize that every woman's experience with her menstrual cycle is unique, and what works for one may not work for another. By encouraging you to listen to your body's cues, such as fatigue, cramps, and bloating, we empower you to make informed decisions about the intensity and duration of your workouts. Whether you choose to ramp up the intensity during high-energy days or dial it back during menstruation, the key is to honor your body and prioritize self-care above all else.

During menstruation, a woman's body undergoes unique changes that can impact her physical and emotional well-being. It's crucial to foster a strong connection with one's body and adapt Wall Pilates practices to individual needs. This involves a nuanced understanding of how intensity and duration play crucial roles in promoting comfort and effectiveness during different phases of the menstrual cycle.

Menstrual Phase (Days 1-5):
- **Intensity:** Consider opting for lower to moderate intensity workouts, respecting the body's need for rest.
- **Duration:** Shorter sessions may be preferred, focusing on gentle movements and stretching to alleviate discomfort.

Follicular Phase (Days 6-14):
- **Intensity:** Gradually increase intensity as energy levels rise, incorporating strength-building exercises.
- **Duration:** Engage in longer sessions, taking advantage of heightened stamina and endurance.

Ovulatory Phase (Days 15-17):
- **Intensity:** Explore moderate to high-intensity workouts, leveraging the peak in energy levels.
- **Duration:** Longer sessions can be well-tolerated, allowing for comprehensive and challenging routines.

Luteal Phase (Days 18-28):
- **Intensity:** Opt for moderate intensity to accommodate potential fatigue and discomfort.
- **Duration:** Focus on maintaining consistency with shorter, well-paced sessions that prioritize flexibility and relaxation.

Adapting Wall Pilates to menstrual cycles involves active communication with the body. Women are encouraged to listen attentively to their energy levels, mood, and any signs of discomfort. This adaptability ensures that each workout remains a positive and empowering experience, contributing to overall health and fitness while nurturing a harmonious relationship with the body's natural rhythms.

<u>**Focus on Gentle Movements, Breathing Techniques, and Nutrition**</u>

In this section, we advocate for a holistic approach to menstrual health that encompasses gentle movements, mindful breathing techniques, and nourishing nutrition. We highlight the benefits of incorporating gentle Pilates movements, such as stretches, pelvic floor exercises, and restorative poses, into your practice to alleviate menstrual symptoms and promote relaxation. Additionally, we explore the role of mindful breathing techniques in reducing stress, enhancing mental clarity, and fostering a sense of calm amidst hormonal fluctuations. Finally, we provide practical nutrition tips for supporting hormonal balance, reducing inflammation, and optimizing menstrual health through whole foods, hydration, and supplementation.

Understanding the intricacies of Wall Pilates during menstruation involves incorporating gentle movements, specific breathing techniques, and mindful nutrition practices. This holistic approach aims to provide comfort, promote relaxation, and support overall well-being during this unique phase of a woman's menstrual cycle.

- **Gentle Movements:** During menstruation, opting for gentle Pilates movements can be highly beneficial. These include:
- **Pelvic Tilts:** Gently engaging the pelvic muscles while lying on the back.
- **Seated Spinal Twist:** A mild twist to alleviate tension in the lower back.
- **Child's Pose:** A restorative posture promoting relaxation and gentle stretching.
- **Breathing Techniques:** Mindful breathing plays a crucial role in enhancing the mind-body connection and managing discomfort. Practices such as:
- **Diaphragmatic Breathing:** Concentrate on taking deep breaths that engage your diaphragm, promoting relaxation throughout your body.
- **Equal Breath:** Inhaling and exhaling for an equal count, fostering a sense of balance and calm.
- **Nutrition Strategies:** Supporting the body with appropriate nutrition is key during menstruation. Consider:
- **Hydration:** Staying well-hydrated to support bodily functions and ease potential bloating.
- **Iron-Rich Foods:** Incorporating iron-rich foods to address potential deficiencies and boost energy.
- **Anti-Inflammatory Foods:** Incorporate foods rich in anti-inflammatory properties into your diet to help alleviate cramps and discomfort during your menstrual cycle.

This chapter emphasizes the synergy between gentle movements, intentional breathing, and mindful nutrition. By tailoring Wall Pilates practices to align with the body's needs during menstruation, women can embrace a holistic approach that nurtures both physical and mental well-being.

Exercises

Day	Focus	Exercise	Description	Duration	Sets/Reps	Suggestions/Notes
1	Awareness and Adaptation	Menstrual Cycle Overview	Understand hormonal changes and energy fluctuations during different menstrual phases.	20 mins	Integrated	Increase self-awareness for adapting Pilates intensity and movements accordingly.
2	Gentle Warm-Up	Pelvic Tilts	Perform gentle pelvic tilts to warm up the lower back and abdominal muscles.	15 mins	3 sets	Focus on smooth, controlled movements to ease tension.
3	Core Stability	Modified Hundreds	Adapt the Hundreds exercise to a comfortable intensity, focusing on core engagement.	20 mins	3 sets	Emphasize breath control and avoid overexertion.
4	Flexibility and Relaxation	Child's Pose with Wall Support	Incorporate the wall for support in Child's Pose, promoting relaxation and flexibility.	15 mins	Integrated	Encourage deep breathing and release tension.
5	Mindful Movement	Seated Meditation with Wall Support	Engage in a seated meditation using the wall for support, promoting mindfulness.	20 mins	Integrated	Focus on calming breathwork and gentle awareness.
6	Full Body Integration	Wall Squats with Pelvic Floor Focus	Perform wall squats with emphasis on engaging the pelvic floor muscles.	20 mins	3 sets	Mindfully integrate pelvic floor engagement into movements.

Understanding Back Pain and its Causes

Back pain is a multifaceted issue that can stem from various sources. Delving deeper into the understanding of back pain and its causes is essential for developing targeted strategies to alleviate discomfort and prevent future issues.

1. Types of Back Pain:
- **Acute Back Pain:** Sudden and intense, usually lasting for a short duration. Often caused by injury or heavy lifting.
- **Chronic Back Pain:** Persistent discomfort lasting for more than three months, often associated with underlying medical conditions.

2. Spinal Anatomy and Back Pain:
- **Vertebrae:** The spine's building blocks, and their misalignment or damage can contribute to pain.
- **Discs:** Act as cushions between vertebrae; herniation or degeneration can cause pain.
- **Muscles and Ligaments:** Strain or tension in these structures can result in back pain.
- **Nerves:** Compression or irritation can lead to radiating pain or sciatica.

3. Lifestyle Factors and Back Pain:
- **Occupational Hazards:** Prolonged sitting, especially with poor ergonomics, can strain the back.
- **Physical Inactivity:** Weak muscles due to lack of exercise contribute to back pain.
- **Poor Posture:** Slouching or maintaining incorrect posture strains the spine.

4. Common Causes of Back Pain:
- **Muscle Strain:** Overexertion, heavy lifting, or sudden movements can strain muscles.
- **Joint Dysfunction:** Misalignment of spinal joints can cause pain and limit mobility.
- **Skeletal Irregularities:** Conditions like scoliosis can contribute to chronic back pain.
- **Diseases:** Conditions like arthritis or osteoporosis may lead to back pain.

5. Contributing Factors:
- **Age:** Degenerative changes in the spine are more common with aging.
- **Weight:** Excess weight puts strain on the spine and can contribute to pain.
- **Psychological Factors:** Stress, anxiety, and depression can manifest as physical back pain.

6. Diagnostic Approaches:
- **Imaging:** MRI, X-rays, or CT scans can identify structural issues.
- **Physical Examination:** Assessing posture, range of motion, and reflexes.
- **Medical History:** Understanding lifestyle, previous injuries, and family history.

7. Prevention and Lifestyle Choices:
- **Exercise:** Regular physical activity strengthens core muscles, supporting the spine.
- **Healthy Weight Management:** Maintaining a healthy weight reduces strain on the spine.
- **Ergonomics:** Proper workplace ergonomics and body mechanics prevent back strain.

8. Seeking Professional Help:
- **Physical Therapy:** Tailored exercises and stretches can alleviate back pain.
- **Medication:** Over the counter or prescription medication may be recommended.
- **Alternative Therapies:** Chiropractic care, acupuncture, or massage can provide relief.

Understanding the complexity of back pain involves recognizing its various forms, pinpointing contributing factors, and adopting a holistic approach to prevention and management. Wall Pilates, with its focus on core strength and flexibility, offers a valuable avenue for individuals seeking to address and mitigate back pain effectively.

Wall Pilates Exercises for Alleviating Back Pain

Day	Focus	Exercise	Description	Duration	Sets/Reps	Suggestions/Notes
1	Core Stability	Wall Plank	Assume a plank position with feet against the wall, engaging core muscles for increased stability.	20 minutes	3 sets of 30s	Engage your core and maintain a neutral spine throughout.
2	Spinal Flexibility and Mobility	Cat-Cow Stretch with Wall Support	Start on hands and knees, use the wall for support while transitioning between arching and rounding.	15 minutes	3 sets of 10	Perform controlled movements, focus on the arching and rounding of the spine.
3	Decompression and stretching	Wall Roll-Downs	Slowly articulate the spine down the wall, engaging core muscles for controlled movement.	20 minutes	3 sets of 12	Move one vertebra at a time, control the descent and ascent.
4	Core Strength and Stability	Wall Teaser	Progress from the floor teaser to a seated position against the wall, engaging core muscles.	20 minutes	Integrated	Engage core muscles, focus on controlled movement.
5	Lateral Core Activation	Wall Side Plank	Engage obliques with a side plank against the wall, lifting hips high and maintaining a straight line.	20 minutes	3 sets of 20s (each side)	Lift hips high, maintain a straight line from head to heels.
6	Lower Back Stretch and Relaxation	Wall Child's Pose	Begin on hands and knees with your feet against the wall, sitting back into a modified child's pose.	15 minutes	1 set of 30s (hold)	Stretch the lower back and encourage relaxation, relieving tension.
7	Spine and Chest Opening	Wall Backbend Stretch	Stand with your back against the wall, arching backward to stretch the front of your body.	15 minutes	1 set of 15-20s (hold)	Open up the chest, stretch the spine, and promote flexibility.
8	Hip Flexor Release	Wall Hip Flexor	Utilize the wall for support while stretching the hip	15 minutes	1 set of 20-30s	Ease tension in the lower back and hip region, enhancing overall

Day	Focus	Exercise	Description	Duration	Sets/Reps	Suggestions/Notes
		Stretch	flexors.		(each side)	back comfort.

Wall Pilates Exercises for a Healthy Back

Day	Area	What	Duration	Duration	Sets/Reps	Suggestions/ Notes
1	Spinal Alignment and Mobility	Wall Cat Stretch	Stand facing the wall, place hands on it, and round your back, then arch it to create a cat stretch.	15 minutes	2 sets of 10	Focus on smooth transitions between rounding and arching the spine.
2	Core Stability	Wall Plank	Assume a plank position with feet against the wall, engaging core muscles for increased stability.	20 minutes	3 sets of 30s	Engage your core and maintain a neutral spine throughout.
3	Decompression and stretching	Wall Roll-Downs	Slowly articulate the spine down the wall, engaging core muscles for controlled movement.	20 minutes	3 sets of 12	Move one vertebra at a time, control the descent and ascent.
4	Pelvic Floor Activation	Wall Bridge	Lie on your back, lift hips toward the ceiling, engaging the pelvic floor and lower back muscles.	20 minutes	3 sets of 15	Squeeze your glutes at the top, keep a steady pace.
5	Lower Back Stretch and Relaxation	Wall Child's Pose	Begin on hands and knees with your feet against the wall, sitting back into a modified child's pose.	15 minutes	1 set of 30s (hold)	Stretch the lower back and encourage relaxation, relieving tension.
6	Lateral Core Activation	Wall Side Plank	Engage obliques with a side plank against the wall, lifting hips high and maintaining a straight line.	20 minutes	3 sets of 20s (each side)	Lift hips high, maintain a straight line from head to heels.
7	Hip Flexor Release	Wall Hip Flexor Stretch	Utilize the wall for support while stretching the hip flexors.	15 minutes	1 set of 20-30s (each side)	Ease tension in the lower back and hip region, enhancing overall back comfort.

Day	Area	What	Duration	Duration	Sets/Reps	Suggestions/ Notes
8	Chest and Shoulder Opening	Wall Chest Opener	Stretch chest muscles by placing hands on the wall and gently leaning forward.	15 minutes	1 set of 15-20s (hold)	Breathe deeply, feel the stretch across the chest.

These exercises are designed to promote a healthy back by focusing on spinal alignment, core stability, flexibility, and targeted muscle activation. Ensure proper form during each exercise and listen to your body. If you have existing back conditions, consult with a healthcare professional before starting a new exercise routine.

Chapter 10: Beyond the Mat - Empowering Your Daily Life

The Mindful Woman: Incorporating Pilates into Daily Activities

In the hustle and bustle of daily life, finding moments of mindfulness can be transformative. This section is dedicated to guiding women on how to seamlessly integrate Pilates principles into their everyday activities. The essence lies in cultivating a mindful approach to movements, breathing, and overall well-being.

Mindfulness in Pilates goes beyond the confines of a workout session. It encourages women to bring conscious awareness to their posture, movements, and breath throughout the day. Whether sitting at a desk, standing in line, or even walking, the principles learned in Pilates can be applied to enhance posture, engage core muscles, and promote overall body awareness.

One key aspect is the incorporation of mindful breathing into daily routines. The breath is a powerful tool in Pilates, and by consciously engaging in deep, diaphragmatic breathing during regular activities, women can experience a sense of calm and centering. This not only fosters physical well-being but also contributes to mental clarity and stress reduction.

Desk-bound professionals, for instance, can integrate simple Pilates-based movements into their work routine. Seated leg lifts, controlled torso twists, or gentle neck stretches can be seamlessly woven into the day to alleviate tension and improve circulation. This not only contributes to physical fitness but also serves as a rejuvenating break for the mind.

Daily chores provide another opportunity for mindful movement. From standing on one leg while doing dishes to maintaining a stable core while carrying groceries, these simple adjustments can turn mundane tasks into mini-Pilates sessions. The emphasis here is on quality movement rather than quantity, fostering a sense of connectivity between mind and body.

For those engaged in regular physical activities such as walking or running, incorporating Pilates principles enhances the effectiveness of these exercises. Emphasis on proper alignment, engaging the core, and controlled breathing can significantly impact the overall quality of the workout, making it more beneficial for the body.

This section provides practical tips and guidance on how to infuse mindfulness into various daily activities. It aims to empower women to view Pilates not just as a scheduled workout but as a holistic approach to living mindfully. By embracing Pilates principles in everyday moments, women can experience the profound impact of this practice on their physical and mental well-being, creating a harmonious integration of Pilates into their daily lives.

Pilates for Women's Health: Addressing Unique Concerns

Chapter 10 delves into the significance of Pilates in addressing the unique health concerns of women. Beyond the mat, Pilates becomes a powerful ally in promoting women's health by specifically targeting areas of concern and fostering overall well-being.

One of the primary focuses is pelvic health. Pilates exercises are designed to engage and strengthen the pelvic floor muscles, crucial for supporting organs, maintaining continence, and addressing issues like pelvic floor dysfunction. By incorporating targeted exercises into their routine, women can take proactive steps in promoting a healthy pelvic floor.

Posture, another key element addressed in this section, plays a pivotal role in women's health. Poor posture can contribute to back pain, neck strain, and other musculoskeletal issues. Pilates, with its emphasis on core strength and alignment, provides women with the tools to improve posture, reducing the risk of associated health issues and promoting a more confident and pain-free lifestyle.

For women going through different life stages, such as pregnancy or menopause, Pilates offers tailored approaches. Similarly, Pilates exercises can help alleviate symptoms associated with menopause, including joint stiffness and decreased bone density.

Breast health is also a consideration in this chapter. Pilates promotes upper body strength and flexibility, contributing to overall breast health. By incorporating exercises that target the chest, shoulders, and upper back, women can enhance muscular support around the breast tissue.

This section emphasizes the role of Pilates in fostering a positive body image and mental well-being. The mind-body connection inherent in Pilates encourages women to appreciate and respect their bodies, promoting a sense of empowerment and self-confidence.

Practical tips, expert insights, and a range of Pilates exercises are provided to address these unique concerns. By understanding and actively engaging in Pilates for women's health, readers can unlock the potential of this practice to enhance their overall quality of life and well-being.

Building Confidence: Embracing Progress and Celebrating Strengths

In Chapter 10, "Beyond the Mat: Empowering Your Daily Life," the focus on building confidence takes center stage. Confidence is not just a state of mind but a holistic aspect of well-being that impacts various facets of life. Pilates, with its transformative powers, becomes a tool for women to enhance their self-assurance, both mentally and physically.

The chapter begins by exploring the psychological benefits of Pilates on confidence. As women engage in mindful movements, they develop a profound connection between their bodies and minds. Pilates encourages a positive mindset, fostering self-love and acceptance. Through intentional breathing and controlled movements, individuals can cultivate a sense of calm and self-assurance that extends beyond the Pilates studio into their daily lives.

The incorporation of progressive routines over the weeks plays a vital role in boosting confidence. By gradually advancing through the exercises, women witness tangible improvements in strength, flexibility, and overall fitness. Small victories in the form of mastering a challenging pose or completing a set contribute to a sense of accomplishment, reinforcing a positive self-image.

Postural improvements, a hallmark of Pilates, also contribute to confidence-building. As women develop core strength and alignment, they naturally carry themselves with better posture. This not only has physical benefits, such as reducing the risk of musculoskeletal issues, but it also positively influences how individuals are perceived by others, further enhancing self-confidence.

The chapter goes on to address the role of Pilates in embracing one's strengths and uniqueness. Rather than adhering to societal ideals, Pilates encourages women to appreciate and celebrate their individual capabilities. This shift in perspective fosters a sense of empowerment, allowing women to embrace their bodies and capabilities with pride.

In addition to physical exercises, the chapter explores the importance of mental well-being in building confidence. Mindfulness techniques and guided meditations are integrated into Pilates sessions to help individuals stay present, release stress, and develop a resilient mindset. This holistic approach ensures that confidence-building extends beyond physical achievements to encompass mental and emotional resilience.

Practical tips, real stories of transformation, and expert guidance are woven into this chapter to provide a comprehensive understanding of how Pilates becomes a powerful ally in building confidence. By the end of the chapter, readers will not only have a repertoire of Pilates exercises but also a newfound sense of empowerment and confidence that permeates every aspect of their lives.

Sustaining Your Practice: A Lifelong Pilates Companion

Sustaining your Pilates practice as a lifelong companion. Pilates is not merely a workout routine; it's a holistic approach to health and well-being that can be integrated into daily life for sustained benefits.

The chapter delves into the strategies and mindset needed to make Pilates a consistent part of one's routine. It emphasizes that Pilates is not a short-term solution but a lifelong journey towards optimal health. By establishing Pilates as a daily habit, individuals can experience continuous improvements in physical fitness, mental well-being, and overall vitality.

To sustain a Pilates practice, the chapter explores the importance of goal setting and creating a personalized plan. Readers are guided on how to set realistic and achievable goals that align with their unique aspirations and lifestyle. Whether the goal is to enhance flexibility, build core strength, or simply enjoy the mental clarity that Pilates brings, having a clear roadmap fosters commitment and motivation.

A crucial aspect of sustaining a Pilates practice is variety. The chapter introduces diverse Pilates routines, ensuring that individuals can adapt their practice to suit their evolving needs and interests. From dynamic workouts to more meditative sessions, the versatility of Pilates allows practitioners to tailor their routines, preventing monotony and keeping the practice enjoyable.

Incorporating Pilates into daily activities is explored as a practical approach to seamlessly integrate the practice into busy schedules. Simple exercises that can be done at home, during work breaks, or while performing daily chores are introduced. This approach reinforces the idea that Pilates is not confined to a specific time or space but can be woven into the fabric of daily life.

To address potential challenges in sustaining a Pilates practice, the chapter provides insights into overcoming common obstacles. Whether it's time constraints, lack of motivation, or external pressures, readers are equipped with strategies to navigate and overcome these hurdles, ensuring that their Pilates journey remains uninterrupted.

Conclusion

Your Pilates Journey—Reflections and Future Steps

As the final chapter of your Pilates guide, the Conclusion serves as a pivotal moment for reflection and contemplation. This chapter encapsulates the essence of the transformative journey readers have undertaken, emphasizing key takeaways, celebrating successes, and charting the course for future steps.

The journey embarked upon by readers is not just a physical one; it's a holistic exploration of mind and body.

Take a moment for a reflective pause: revisit the initial motivations that led you to Wall Pilates.

This was a deeper understanding of personal growth, accomplishments, and the evolving relationship with your body.

Congratulation for your resilience and commitment! Whether it was dispelling myths, building confidence, addressing specific circumstances like pregnancy or menstruation, or overcoming back issues, each obstacle conquered is a testament to the strength cultivated through Pilates.

Think about the interconnectedness of physical and mental well-being! Pilates extends beyond a series of exercises—it's a philosophy that integrates breath, movement, and mindfulness.

Reflect on the mental and emotional shifts experienced during the journey, recognizing the symbiotic relationship between a strong, agile body and a calm, focused mind.

To further enrich the reflective process, document your personal reflections. Whether through journaling, goal setting, or creating a visual representation of your Pilates journey, this exercise solidifies the impact of the guide on an individual level.

Take ownership of your progresses, well done!

Now read a practical guidance on how you can continue your Pilates journey independently. There are recommendations for ongoing routines, tips for incorporating Pilates into evolving fitness goals, and suggestions for further education or exploration within the realm of Pilates.

The importance of community: share your experiences, connect with fellow practitioners, and celebrate collective achievements. This sense of community contributes to the sustainability of the Pilates journey, fostering motivation and a shared commitment to lifelong well-being.

Please note that Pilates is not merely a 28-day challenge but a lifelong companion in the pursuit of optimal health and vitality!

Personal Reflections and Success Stories: Chronicles of Transformation

This section within the Conclusion is dedicated to capturing the individual narratives that have unfolded throughout the Pilates journey. It's a tapestry of personal reflections and success stories—testimonials to the transformative power of Wall Pilates. As readers engage in introspection, recounting their unique experiences, they contribute to a collective narrative that echoes the diverse and profound impact of this holistic practice.

The power of personal reflection lies in its ability to unveil the subtle shifts that occur within. It prompts individuals to revisit the initial motives that propelled them onto this Pilates odyssey. Readers are encouraged to ponder not only the physical changes—a stronger core, increased flexibility, or enhanced balance—but also the less tangible, yet equally significant, mental, and emotional transformations.

Success stories serve as beacons of inspiration, illuminating the path for others to follow. In this deep dive into Personal Reflections and Success Stories, the chapter sheds light on the multifaceted nature of success. It goes beyond numerical achievements or outward physical changes, delving into the stories of individuals who found solace in Pilates during challenging times, experienced heightened self-awareness, or forged connections with their bodies in ways they hadn't imagined.

Readers are invited to express their triumphs, both big and small. Whether it's conquering a challenging Pilates pose, staying committed to the 28-day workout challenge, or experiencing a profound mental shift during meditation, each success story contributes to the rich tapestry of this Pilates community.

The deep dive into personal reflections involves providing prompts and exercises that guide readers through a structured self-inquiry. Journaling becomes a powerful tool for self-discovery, enabling individuals to articulate their thoughts, emotions, and realizations. This section prompts readers to explore how Pilates has influenced their daily lives, relationships, and overall well-being.

Intertwined with these personal reflections are snippets of success stories shared by individuals who have embraced the Pilates journey. These narratives are diverse, touching upon various aspects such as increased body confidence, enhanced focus, and the joy of achieving milestones previously deemed unattainable.

The narrative also explores the role of the Pilates community in shaping these personal reflections and success stories. It highlights the supportive and encouraging environment cultivated by practitioners, emphasizing the notion that the collective journey is as integral as the individual paths.

In essence, this deep dive into Personal Reflections and Success Stories transcends the confines of a fitness guide. It becomes a testament to the profound impact that mindful movement, intentional breath, and the practice of Pilates can have on the lives of individuals. As readers share their stories and reflections, they contribute not only to the conclusion of this guide but also to the ongoing narrative of empowerment, growth, and well-being within the Pilates community.

Success Story 1: Empowering Core Strength

Sarah's journey into the world of Wall Pilates began with a desire for a holistic fitness routine that extended beyond the conventional gym experience. As a corporate professional juggling the demands of a high-pressure job, Sarah sought a form of exercise that not only promised physical benefits but also provided a mental and emotional escape.

Upon discovering the dedicated focus on core strength within the 28-day Wall Pilates challenge, Sarah was intrigued. The Core Stability exercises, meticulously designed for beginners like her, aimed at building a strong foundation. Wall Planks, Wall Crunches, and Wall Bridges became integral parts of her daily practice. The initial days brought challenges, but Sarah persisted, guided by the detailed instructions and suggestions provided in the daily workout routine.

One of the key milestones in Sarah's journey was mastering the Wall Plank. The position, with feet against the wall, added an extra dimension to the traditional plank, intensifying the engagement of core muscles. The 20 minutes dedicated to this exercise, divided into 3 sets of 30 seconds each, became a ritual that she looked forward to.

The Wall Crunches, performed with controlled movements and utilizing the wall for support, targeted the abdominal muscles. Sarah learned to focus on precision, avoiding strain on her neck and ensuring that each movement contributed to the strengthening of her core.

The Wall Bridge exercise added a dynamic element to her routine. Lying on her back, Sarah lifted her hips toward the ceiling, engaging her core and squeezing her glutes at the top. This exercise not only targeted the core but also worked on lower body strength.

Throughout the journey, Sarah embraced the guidance to maintain a neutral spine, control movements, and pay attention to breathing patterns. The comprehensive approach of the Wall Pilates program, combining strength-building with mindfulness, resonated with her overarching goal of achieving a harmonious balance in her physical and mental well-being.

As Sarah progressed through the 28-day challenge, she not only experienced a noticeable improvement in her core strength but also felt a transformative shift in her overall confidence. The stability gained through Wall Pilates became a metaphor for the stability she sought in her demanding professional life.

By the end of the challenge, Sarah had not just unlocked a stronger core but also discovered a newfound self-assurance that extended beyond the walls of her Pilates space. This success story highlights the empowering journey of a woman who, through the dedicated practice of Wall Pilates, not only transformed her physical strength but also cultivated a deeper connection between her body and mind. Sarah's story stands as a testament to the transformative powers of Wall Pilates, making it not just an exercise routine but a journey toward self-discovery and empowerment.

Success Story 2: Building Confidence Through Wall Pilates

Meet Emily, a woman in her mid-30s who embarked on her Wall Pilates journey seeking a fitness routine that would not only sculpt her body but also boost her confidence. Emily had tried various workout programs, but they often left her feeling overwhelmed or discouraged.

Upon discovering the 28-day Wall Pilates challenge, Emily was intrigued by its progressive approach. The program promised not just physical transformation but also a focus on building confidence. Week 1, dedicated to foundational exercises, provided Emily with a gentle introduction to the world of Wall Pilates.

The daily routine began with Core Stability exercises, including the Wall Plank, Wall Crunches, and Wall Bridge. These exercises, aimed at strengthening the core muscles, allowed Emily to start at her own pace. The detailed instructions and suggestions provided in the program ensured that she maintained proper form and gradually increased the intensity.

As Week 2 unfolded with a focus on Upper Body Strengthening, Emily found herself challenged in a positive way. Wall Push-Ups, Wall Tricep Dips, and Wall Arm Circles became integral parts of her routine. The emphasis on controlled movements and maintaining a straight line from head to heels during push-ups helped Emily build strength in her arms and chest.

The Lower Body Activation exercises in Week 3, such as Wall Squats, Wall Leg Raises, and Wall Side Leg Lifts, brought a new dimension to Emily's workout. These exercises not only targeted her lower body but also improved her overall stability and balance.

Week 4, with a focus on Flexibility and Stretching, provided Emily with a well-rounded conclusion to the 28-day challenge. The integration of dynamic Pilates movements and fusion exercises, such as Wall Roll-Downs, Wall Scissor Kicks, and Wall Pike, challenged her body in new ways. The slow articulation of the spine and controlled movements in each exercise contributed to both flexibility and strength.

Throughout the 28 days, Emily not only witnessed a positive transformation in her physical appearance but also felt a significant boost in her confidence. The progressive nature of the program allowed her to overcome initial doubts and plateaus, building a sense of accomplishment with each passing week.

By the end of the challenge, Emily not only felt more physically fit but also carried herself with a newfound confidence in her daily life. This success story illustrates the transformative power of Wall Pilates in not just shaping the body but also instilling a sense of confidence and self-assurance in women like Emily, making it a holistic approach to fitness and well-being.

Success Story 3: Empowering Mind and Body Through Wall Pilates

Meet Sarah, a busy professional in her late 20s who, like many others, struggled to find a fitness routine that accommodated her hectic schedule. Sarah was not only looking for physical benefits but also sought a way to alleviate stress and improve her mental well-being.

Upon discovering the 28-day Wall Pilates challenge, Sarah was drawn to its holistic approach, combining physical exercises with mindful movements. As someone who spent long hours at a desk, Sarah appreciated the emphasis on the mind-body connection that Wall Pilates promotes.

During Week 1, as the program focused on Core Stability exercises, Sarah found herself engaged in exercises like the Wall Plank, Wall Crunches, and Wall Bridge. The incorporation of breathwork and mindful movements helped her not only strengthen her core but also develop a sense of awareness in her body.

Week 2, dedicated to Upper Body Strengthening, introduced Sarah to Wall Push-Ups, Wall Tricep Dips, and Wall Arm Circles. The controlled movements and intentional focus required in these exercises allowed Sarah to channel her energy positively. The gradual progression in difficulty kept her motivated, and she felt a noticeable improvement in her upper body strength.

Lower Body Activation exercises in Week 3, including Wall Squats, Wall Leg Raises, and Wall Side Leg Lifts, brought a sense of balance and stability to Sarah's routine. The integration of mindfulness in these movements allowed her to connect with her body on a deeper level, fostering a sense of well-being.

Week 4, with a focus on Flexibility and Stretching, resonated with Sarah's desire for stress relief. The Wall Pilates movements, such as Wall Roll-Downs, Wall Scissor Kicks, and Wall Pike, became not just physical exercises but moments of mental relaxation. The mind-body fusion in these exercises contributed to Sarah's overall emotional and mental wellness.

Beyond the 28-day challenge, Sarah discovered that Wall Pilates had become more than just a workout routine—it became her daily escape. The mindful approach to movement helped her manage stress, and the physical benefits were complemented by a newfound mental clarity.

This success story highlights the transformative power of Wall Pilates in not only sculpting the body but also fostering a positive connection between mind and body. For busy individuals like Sarah, Wall Pilates offered a holistic wellness solution that transcended the boundaries of traditional fitness, making it a sustainable and enriching part of her daily life.

Success Story 4: Rediscovering Strength and Confidence with Wall Pilates

Meet Emily, a woman in her early 40s who, after a hiatus from regular exercise, found herself yearning to regain strength and confidence in her body. Juggling the demands of a full-time job and family life, Emily sought a fitness routine that was not only effective but also accommodating to her busy schedule.

Upon discovering the Wall Pilates program, Emily was intrigued by its emphasis on gradual progression and its accessibility to all fitness levels. The 28-day challenge seemed like the perfect starting point for someone reacquainting themselves with fitness.

During Week 1, the focus on Core Stability exercises introduced Emily to fundamental movements like the Wall Plank, Wall Crunches, and Wall Bridge. The controlled and supportive nature of these exercises provided a gentle reentry into physical activity, allowing Emily to rebuild her core strength without feeling overwhelmed.

Week 2, dedicated to Upper Body Strengthening, became a turning point for Emily. With exercises such as Wall Push-Ups, Wall Tricep Dips, and Wall Arm Circles, she felt a gradual but noticeable improvement in her upper body strength. The use of the wall for support made these exercises approachable, even for someone who had been away from regular workouts.

Lower Body Activation in Week 3, featuring Wall Squats, Wall Leg Raises, and Wall Side Leg Lifts, helped Emily reconnect with her lower body muscles. The supportive environment of the wall allowed her to focus on form and control, building a strong foundation for future workouts.

By Week 4, with a focus on Flexibility and Stretching, Emily felt a sense of accomplishment and increased confidence. Movements like Wall Roll-Downs, Wall Scissor Kicks, and Wall Pike not only improved her flexibility but also contributed to a positive mindset about her body's capabilities.

Beyond the 28-day challenge, Emily discovered a newfound appreciation for regular physical activity. Wall Pilates became her go-to workout, seamlessly fitting into her daily routine. The progressive nature of the program allowed her to challenge herself at her own pace, contributing to a sustainable and enjoyable fitness journey.

This success story underscores the empowering nature of Wall Pilates for individuals like Emily, who may have taken a break from regular exercise. Through a combination of accessible movements, gradual progression, and a supportive environment, Emily not only regained physical strength but also discovered a renewed sense of confidence in her body and its capabilities.

Appendix

BOOK Summary

As you embark on your Wall Pilates journey, understanding the terminology is key to maximizing your practice. This comprehensive glossary provides definitions for essential terms used throughout the book, ensuring clarity and empowering you to fully engage with the transformative powers of Wall Pilates.

Wall Pilates:
A unique style of Pilates integrating the support and resistance of a wall, fostering improved stability, balance, and heightened body awareness.

Core Principles:
The foundational concepts that underpin Wall Pilates, emphasizing core engagement, breath control, and mindful movement.

Mind-Body Connection:
The awareness of the relationship between your mental and physical states, central to the practice of Wall Pilates.

Guided Meditation:
A focused mental exercise that promotes relaxation and enhances the mind-body connection, often integrated into Wall Pilates sessions.

Foundation Fitness Assessment: - A series of tests to evaluate flexibility, strength, balance, and other fitness parameters, helping tailor Wall Pilates routines to individual needs.

28-Day Wall Pilates Workout Challenge: - A structured four-week program designed to progressively enhance strength, flexibility, and overall fitness through daily Wall Pilates exercises.

Wall Pilates Confidence Builder: - The initial phase of the 28-day challenge focusing on foundational exercises to build confidence and familiarity with Wall Pilates.

Overcoming Plateaus and Challenges: - The second phase of the 28-day challenge targeting more advanced exercises to push beyond initial limits and enhance overall fitness.

Safe Wall Pilates Practices for Expectant Mothers: - Guidelines and exercises tailored for pregnant individuals to safely practice Wall Pilates and support overall well-being during pregnancy.

Adapting Routines for Different Pregnancy Stages: - Modifying Wall Pilates exercises based on the trimester to accommodate the changing needs and comfort levels of expectant mothers.

Understanding Menstrual Changes and Exercise: - Insights into how menstrual cycles may impact energy levels and exercise performance, guiding modifications for a comfortable Wall Pilates practice.

Listening to Your Body: Modifying Intensity and Duration: - The practice of tuning into bodily signals during menstruation and adjusting Wall Pilates intensity and duration accordingly for a supportive experience.

Focus on Gentle Movements, Breathing Techniques, and Nutrition: - Emphasizing gentle Wall Pilates movements, mindful breathing, and nutritional considerations to enhance comfort and well-being during menstruation.

Addressing Common Concerns with Real Stories from Women: - Providing practical solutions and insights into common concerns related to Wall Pilates during menstruation, accompanied by real stories from women who have navigated these challenges.

Understanding Back Pain and its Causes: - Exploring the factors contributing to back pain and how Wall Pilates can be utilized to alleviate discomfort and promote a healthy back.

Wall Pilates Exercises for a Healthy Back: - Specific exercises targeting back strength, flexibility, and alignment to support a healthy spine and reduce the risk of back pain.

The Mindful Woman: Incorporating Pilates into Daily Activities: - A holistic approach to mindfulness, encouraging the integration of Pilates principles into everyday activities for enhanced body awareness and well-being.

Sustaining Your Practice: A Lifelong Pilates Companion: - Guidance on incorporating Wall Pilates into a lifelong wellness journey, emphasizing sustainability and ongoing commitment for enduring health benefits.

This glossary serves as a valuable resource, ensuring you have a clear understanding of the language surrounding Wall Pilates, empowering you to fully immerse yourself in this transformative practice.

<u>GLOSSARY: Step by step description of all the Exercises</u>

GLOSSARY	
Exercise	**Step by Step Description**
Wall Squats	Position yourself with your back against the wall and your feet spaced hip-width apart Descend into a squat while ensuring your back remains in contact with the wall and your knees align with your ankles. Hold the squat position for a few seconds, then return to the starting position. Repeat for the desired number of repetitions.
Wall glute bridge	Lie on your back with your feet flat against the wall, hip-width apart and knees bent. Push against the wall with your feet as you elevate your hips towards the ceiling, engaging your glutes and core musclesTop of Form Hold the bridge position at the top for a moment. Next, gently lower your hips back to the initial position, maintaining control and stability throughout the movement. Maintain a neutral spine throughout the exercise, being mindful not to arch your lower back excessively. This helps to protect your spine and engage the core muscles effectively For added challenge, you can perform single-leg glute bridges by lifting one foot off the wall at a time.
Wall Side Lunges (Left)	Stand facing the wall with your feet together and arms at your sides. Take a wide step out to the side with your left foot, bending your left knee and shifting your weight towards it as you lower into a lunge. Keep your right leg straight and your chest lifted as you lower down, reaching your left hand towards the wall for support. Push through the heel of your left foot to return to the initial standing position. This action engages the muscles of the left leg and promotes stability and balance
Wall Side Lunges (right)	Stand facing the wall with your feet together and arms at your sides. Take a wide step out to the side with your right foot, bending your left knee and shifting your weight towards it as you lower into a lunge. Keep your left leg straight and your chest lifted as you lower down, reaching your left hand towards the wall for support. Push through the heel of your left foot to return to the initial standing position. This action engages the muscles of the left leg and promotes stability and balance

GLOSSARY	
Exercise	**Step by Step Description**
Wall Push Ups	Begin in a push-up position facing towards the wall, with your hands placed slightly wider than shoulder-width apart and arms fully extended. Activate your core muscles and ensure your body forms a straight line from your head to your heels, maintaining a neutral spine position. This helps stabilize your body and supports proper alignment during the exercise. Bend your elbows and lower your chest towards the wall, keeping them close to your body as you descend. Use your palms to exert force and lift your body back to the initial position, fully extending your arms. Continue the exercise for the desired number of repetitions, ensuring that you maintain proper form and execute each movement with control. Consistency in maintaining proper technique is crucial for maximizing the effectiveness of the exercise and preventing injury.
Wall Diamond Push Ups	Stand facing the wall with your feet hip-width apart and your hands placed flat against the wall at shoulder width, forming a diamond shape with your thumbs and index fingers. Walk your feet back a few steps until your body is at a slight angle, with your arms fully extended and your hands supporting your weight. Activate your core muscles and gradually lower your chest towards the wall by flexing your elbows, ensuring they remain near your torso throughout the movement. This targets the muscles in your arms and chest while maintaining stability in your core.. Descend until your chest nearly reaches the wall, ensuring controlled movement, then exert force through your palms to return to the initial position. This exercise effectively engages your upper body muscles while promoting stability and control. Keep your body in a straight line from head to heels throughout the movement, maintaining tension in your core and glutes for stability. Perform the push-up movement for the designated number of reps, prioritizing form and control throughout. This exercise targets your upper body strength while emphasizing stability and precision with each repetition.
Wall Shoulder Taps	Begin in a plank position facing the wall, with your hands placed shoulder-width apart on the wall and your body forming a straight line from head to heels. Engage your core muscles to stabilize your torso and Ensure to avoid excessive movement or sagging in the lower back throughout the exercise. Elevate your left hand away from the wall and gently touch your right shoulder with it, then smoothly bring it back to its initial position against the wall. Repeat the movement with your right hand, tapping your left shoulder. Continue alternating shoulder taps while maintaining a strong plank position and minimizing any rotation or sway in your hips. Aim to tap each shoulder for the desired number of repetitions, focusing on controlled movement and stability throughout.
Wall standing knee drives	Stand facing the wall with your feet hip-width apart and your arms extended overhead, palms flat against the wall. Engage your core muscles to stabilize your torso and maintain balance. Lift your left knee towards your chest, driving it up towards the wall as high as possible while keeping your chest lifted. Lower your left foot back to the ground and immediately drive your right knee up towards the wall in a fluid, continuous motion. Continue alternating knee drives, focusing on driving your knees up towards the wall with control and precision. Maintain a steady pace and rhythm throughout the exercise, aiming for the desired number of repetitions on each leg.

GLOSSARY	
Exercise	**Step by Step Description**
Wall Cross Body Crunches	Stand facing the wall with your feet hip-width apart and your back flat against the wall. Extend your arms straight out in front of you and place your palms flat against the wall at shoulder height. Engage your core muscles and lift your right knee up towards your chest, bringing it across your body towards your left elbow. At the same time, twist your torso to the left, bringing your right elbow towards your right knee in a cross-body motion. Contract your abdominal muscles as you crunch, squeezing your obliques to bring your knee and elbow as close together as possible. Slowly return to the starting position, extending your right leg back down to the ground and straightening your torso. Repeat the movement on the opposite side, lifting your left knee towards your right elbow and twisting your torso to the right. Continue alternating sides, performing controlled and deliberate movements to target the obliques and core muscles effectively.
Wall Reach Through Crunches	Lie on your back with your legs extended straight up towards the ceiling, pressing your feet against the wall. Extend your arms overhead and reach towards the wall, engaging your core muscles to lift your head, neck, and shoulders off the ground. Crunch upwards, reaching your hands towards your feet as if trying to touch the wall. Lower your upper body back down with control, keeping your lower back pressed into the ground. Repeat the crunching motion, focusing on engaging your abdominals and maintaining a smooth, controlled movement pattern. Aim to reach towards the wall with each repetition, maximizing the range of motion and targeting your abdominal muscles effectively.
Wall Sit with Leg Extensions	Start by standing with your back against the wall and your feet hip-width apart. Lower yourself into a seated position, sliding your back down the wall until your thighs are parallel to the ground. Hold this position, engaging your core and pressing your lower back into the wall for support. Extend your right leg straight out in front of you, keeping it parallel to the ground. Hold the leg extension for a few seconds, then return your right foot to the ground. Repeat the leg extension on the left side, alternating legs for the desired number of repetitions. Focus on maintaining proper posture and keeping your core engaged throughout the exercise.
Wall Glute Kickbacks (Right)	Stand facing the wall with your feet hip-width apart and your hands resting lightly against the wall for support. Shift your weight onto your left leg and lift your right knee up towards your chest, keeping your core engaged for balance. Extend your right leg straight back behind you, pressing through your heel to engage your glutes and lift your leg as high as possible. Keep your hips square to the wall and avoid arching your lower back as you extend your leg. Pause at the top of the movement, squeezing your glutes to maximize the contraction in your right buttock. Slowly lower your right leg back down to the starting position, returning to a standing position with both feet on the ground. Repeat the movement for the desired number of repetitions, then switch to the opposite side to perform the exercise with your left leg.

GLOSSARY

Exercise	Step by Step Description
Wall Glute Kickbacks (Left)	Start by standing facing away from the wall, with your hands resting lightly against the wall for support. Shift your weight onto your right leg and lift your left foot off the ground, bending your left knee at a 90-degree angle. Exhale as you extend your left leg straight back behind you, squeezing your left glute at the top of the movement. Inhale as you bend your left knee and return your left foot to the starting position. Perform the same kickback movement on your left side, ensuring controlled movements and engaging your glute muscles throughout the exercise. Aim for a full range of motion while maintaining stability and balance.
Wall Tricep Press	Stand facing the wall with your feet hip-width apart and your palms pressed flat against the wall at shoulder height. Lean your body weight into the wall, keeping your elbows close to your sides and your upper arms parallel to the ground. Engage your triceps as you press your palms into the wall, straightening your arms. Hold the press for a moment, then slowly bend your elbows to lower your body towards the wall. Keep your core engaged and avoid arching your back during the movement. Return to the starting position by pressing back up, and repeat the exercise for the desired number of repetitions.
Wall Arm Angels	Stand with your back against the wall and arms extended out to the sides at shoulder height. Slowly raise your arms overhead, keeping them in contact with the wall. Lower your arms back down to shoulder height, maintaining contact with the wall throughout the movement. Repeat for the desired number of repetitions.
Wall Thread the Needle	Kneeling in front of the wall with knees hips width and hands slightly against the wall for support. Extend your arms straight out in front of you and place your palms flat against the wall at shoulder height. Engage your core muscles and lift your right knee up towards your chest, bringing it across your body towards your left elbow. Rotate your torso to the left as you lift your right knee, allowing your right hip to open up and your knee to point towards the left side of your body. Thread your right leg under your body and through the space between your left leg and left arm, aiming to touch your right foot to the ground on the left side of your body. Keep your core engaged and your back straight as you rotate and twist through the movement, feeling a stretch in your lower back and hips. Return to the starting position by reversing the movement, lifting your right knee back up towards your chest and rotating your torso to the right. Repeat the movement for the desired number of repetitions, then switch to the opposite side to perform the exercise with your left leg.
Wall Plank	Begin by facing the wall in a standing position, arms extended at shoulder height and palms flat against the wall. Walk your feet back until your body forms a straight line from head to heels, supported by your arms. Engage your core muscles to maintain stability and hold this position for the desired duration. Keep your neck neutral and avoid sagging or arching your lower back. To modify, you can perform the plank on your forearms instead of your hands.

<table>
<tr><th colspan="2">GLOSSARY</th></tr>
<tr><th>Exercise</th><th>Step by Step Description</th></tr>
<tr><td>Wall Toe Touch Crunches</td><td>Stand facing the wall with your feet hip-width apart and your arms extended straight up towards the ceiling.
Engage your core muscles and slightly bend your knees as you hinge forward at the hips, reaching your fingertips towards your toes.
Exhale as you lift your legs off the ground, bringing your knees towards your chest while simultaneously bringing your torso towards your thighs.
Keep your abdominal muscles engaged throughout the movement to control the descent.
Inhale as you lower your legs back down towards the ground, extending them straight out in front of you.
Continue performing the exercise for the designated number of repetitions, ensuring that you maintain proper form and control with each repetition.</td></tr>
<tr><td>Wall Elevated Plank Side Steps</td><td>Begin in an elevated plank position facing the wall, with your hands flat against the wall at shoulder height and slightly wider than shoulder-width apart.
Engage your core muscles to keep your body in a straight line from head to heels, with your hips level and your feet together.
Maintaining this plank position, take small side steps to the right by moving your right hand and foot together, followed by your left hand and foot.
Ensure that your movements are controlled and deliberate, emphasizing stability and balance throughout the exercise.
After completing several steps to the right, reverse direction and take side steps to the left, leading with your left hand and foot.
Continue alternating side steps to the right and left, moving at a pace that challenges your balance and coordination while maintaining proper form.</td></tr>
<tr><td>Wall Walking Glute Bridge</td><td>Begin by lying on your back on the floor with your feet flat against the wall and your knees bent at a 90-degree angle.
Press your feet into the wall as you lift your hips towards the ceiling, driving through your heels to engage your glutes and hamstrings.
Once your hips are fully lifted into a bridge position, slowly walk your feet up the wall one at a time, inching your way higher towards the ceiling.
Continue walking your feet up the wall until your legs are extended straight and your body forms a straight line from shoulders to heels.
Hold the elevated bridge position at the top for a moment, then reverse the movement by walking your feet back down the wall to return to the starting position.
Focus on maintaining control and stability throughout the exercise, keeping your core engaged and your hips lifted throughout the movement.</td></tr>
<tr><td>Wall Pilates 100's</td><td>Lie on your back with your legs extended straight up towards the ceiling, forming a 90-degree angle with your torso.
Lift your head, neck, and shoulders off the ground, reaching your arms straight towards your feet.
Initiate small, controlled movements by pumping your arms up and down while synchronizing your breath. Inhale deeply for a count of five, then exhale for another count of five. Repeat this pattern throughout the exercise.
Continue pumping your arms rhythmically as you maintain the lifted position and engage your core muscles.
Aim to complete 100 arm pumps while keeping your legs and torso stable and your lower back pressed into the ground.</td></tr>
<tr><td>Wall plank to pike</td><td>This is a difficult exercise. It's better to see the Video via Qr Code to understand the details</td></tr>
<tr><td>Wall Single Leg Glute Bridge (Right)</td><td>Target one leg at a time with single-leg glute bridge against the wall.
Start by lying on your back with your feet flat against the wall and your knees bent.
Extend your right leg straight up towards the ceiling, pressing your heel into the wall.
Engage your left foot firmly against the ground as you lift your hips upwards, focusing on squeezing your glutes at the peak of the movement.</td></tr>
</table>

GLOSSARY	
Exercise	**Step by Step Description**
	Keep your hips level and avoid rotating or tilting to one side. With control, lower your hips back down to the starting position and repeat the movement for the desired number of repetitions. Focus on maintaining proper form and controlled movement throughout.
Wall Single Leg Glute Bridge (Left)	Target one leg at a time with single-leg glute bridge against the wall. Start by lying on your back with your feet flat against the wall and your knees bent. Extend your left leg straight up towards the ceiling, pressing your heel into the wall. Press through your right foot to lift your hips off the ground, squeezing your glutes at the top of the movement. Keep your hips level and avoid rotating or tilting to one side. With control, lower your hips back down to the starting position and repeat the movement for the desired number of repetitions. Focus on maintaining proper form and controlled movement throughout.
Wall plie squats	Stand facing the wall with your feet wider than hip-width apart and your toes turned out at a comfortable angle. Place your hands on the wall for support, keeping your arms extended straight out in front of you at shoulder height. Engage your core muscles and lower your body down towards the ground, bending your knees and keeping them aligned with your toes. Keep your chest lifted and your back straight as you lower into the squat position, aiming to bring your thighs parallel to the ground. Press through your heels to push yourself back up to the starting position, fully extending your legs and returning to standing. Continue to perform the exercise for the prescribed number of repetitions, concentrating on maintaining correct form and control throughout each repetition.
Wall Diamonds	This is an important exercise. Please see the Video via Qr Code to understand the details
Wall Commando Planks	Start in a plank position facing away from the wall, with your hands on the ground directly under your shoulders and your feet against the wall. Lower yourself down onto your forearms one arm at a time, maintaining a straight body line. Return to the initial plank position by pushing up with one arm at a time. Repeat for the desired number of repetitions.
Wall Arm Butterflies	This is an important exercise. Please see the Video via Qr Code to understand the details
Wall Elevated Plank	This is an important exercise. Please see the Video via Qr Code to understand the details
Wall Lying Hip Adductions	Lie on your back on the floor with your legs extended straight up against the wall, forming a 90-degree angle with your hips and knees. Place your arms by your sides or extend them out to the sides for balance. Engage your core muscles and press your lower back into the floor to stabilize your pelvis. Keeping your legs straight, slowly lower them out to the sides as far as comfortably possible, feeling a stretch in your inner thighs. Use your inner thigh muscles to bring your legs back together, squeezing them towards the midline of your body. Repeat the movement for the desired number of repetitions, focusing on maintaining control and stability throughout.
Wall Single Arm Tricep Press (Right)	Stand facing the wall with your feet hip-width apart and your right side closest to the wall. Place your right hand against the wall at shoulder height, with your elbow bent and your palm facing down. Engage your core muscles and press your palm into the wall to straighten your arm, focusing on squeezing your triceps. Maintain proper form by keeping your elbow close to your body throughout the movement. Avoid swinging or making excessive movements to ensure you target the intended muscles effectivel.

Exercise	Step by Step Description
	Slowly bend your elbow to lower your body back towards the wall, feeling a stretch in your triceps. Repeat the movement for the desired number of repetitions, then switch sides to perform the exercise with your left arm
Wall Reverse Lunges	Stand facing away from the wall with your feet hip-width apart and your arms by your sides. Step backward with your right foot, ensuring both knees are bent at 90-degree angles as you lower your body toward the ground. Maintain proper form and control throughout the movement. Keep your chest lifted and your back straight as you lower into the lunge position, aiming to bring your back knee towards the ground without touching it. Press through your left heel to push yourself back up to the starting position, fully extending your legs and returning to standing. Alternate legs with each repetition, stepping back with your left foot to repeat the movement on the opposite side. Continue alternating reverse lunges for the desired number of repetitions, focusing on maintaining proper form and control throughout.
Wall Side to Side Lunges	Stand facing the wall with your feet together and your hands on your hips or extended out in front of you for balance. Take a wide step to the right with your right foot, bending your right knee and lowering your body into a side lunge position. Keep your left leg straight and your left foot flat on the ground as you lower your hips towards the wall, maintaining a neutral spine and engaging your core. Once you reach the bottom of the lunge, press through your right heel to push yourself back up to the starting position, returning to standing. Alternate legs with each repetition, stepping back with your left foot to repeat the movement on the opposite side. Continue alternating side lunges to the right and left, moving at a controlled pace and focusing on maintaining proper form throughout the exercise. This exercise targets the muscles of the lower body, including the quadriceps, hamstrings, glutes, and adductors, while also improving hip mobility and stability.

Fueling Your Wall Pilates Journey: A Comprehensive Nutrition Guide for Maximum Results

Embarking on your Wall Pilates journey involves more than just mastering poses and building strength; it requires a holistic approach to well-being. Nutrition plays a vital role in supporting your body through the demands of Wall Pilates, promoting energy, recovery, and overall health. In this comprehensive guide, we'll delve into key nutritional principles, meal planning strategies, and hydration practices tailored to maximize your Wall Pilates experience.

Foundations of Nutrition for Wall Pilates:

1. Nutrient-Rich Whole Foods:

Prioritize a diet rich in whole foods, including fruits, vegetables, lean proteins, whole grains, and healthy fats. These nutrient-dense choices provide essential vitamins and minerals for overall health.

2. Balanced Macronutrients:

Aim for a balanced intake of macronutrients—carbohydrates, proteins, and fats. Carbohydrates provide energy, proteins support muscle repair, and healthy fats contribute to overall well-being.

3. Adequate Protein Intake:

Protein is crucial for muscle repair and recovery. Ensure a sufficient intake of lean protein sources like poultry, fish, beans, and tofu. Consider incorporating protein into each meal to support your body's needs.

4. Mindful Eating:

Practice mindful eating by paying attention to hunger and fullness cues. Avoid distractions during meals, savor each bite, and listen to your body's signals to maintain a healthy relationship with food.

Meal Planning Strategies:

1. Pre-Workout Nutrition:

Fueling your body before a Wall Pilates session is essential. Consume a balanced meal containing carbohydrates, proteins, and a small amount of healthy fats 2-3 hours before exercising. This provides sustained energy and supports muscle function.

2. Post-Workout Recovery:

Optimize recovery by consuming a post-workout meal or snack rich in protein and carbohydrates. This pairing aids in replenishing glycogen stores and facilitating muscle repair. Examples include a protein smoothie, Greek yogurt with fruit, or a chicken and vegetable stir-fry.

3. Hydration as a Foundation:

Hydration is key for overall well-being and performance. Start your day with water, stay hydrated throughout, and incorporate water-rich foods like cucumbers and watermelon into your meals. Adjust your water intake based on activity levels and environmental conditions.

4. Snacking for Sustained Energy:

Include nutritious snacks in your daily routine to maintain energy levels between meals. Opt for options like nuts, seeds, Greek yogurt, or fruit to support stable blood sugar levels and prevent energy dips.

5. Whole Foods for Nutrient Density:

Choose whole, minimally processed foods to maximize nutrient density. These foods provide a broad spectrum of vitamins, minerals, and antioxidants that contribute to overall health and vitality.

Hydration Strategies for Optimal Performance:

1. Water Intake Timing:

Distribute water intake throughout the day, starting with a glass in the morning. Keep a water bottle within reach and sip consistently to stay adequately hydrated.

2. Pre-Workout Hydration:

Consume 16-20 ounces of water 2-3 hours before your Wall Pilates session to ensure proper hydration and support optimal performance.

3. During Exercise Hydration:

Sip water during breaks, considering the intensity and duration of your workout. While Pilates may not induce heavy sweating, maintaining consistent hydration is essential.

4. Post-Workout Rehydration:

Rehydrate after your session, especially if it was intense or prolonged. Consider adding a pinch of salt to your water to support electrolyte balance.

5. Monitor Urine Color:

Observe the color of your urine as a straightforward gauge of your hydration level. Aim for pale yellow urine, suggesting adequate hydration.

Individualized Approach:

1. Adjusting to Unique Needs:

Recognize that everyone's nutritional needs are unique. Factors such as body weight, activity levels, and personal preferences influence dietary requirements. Experiment and tailor your nutrition to what works best for you.

2. Listen to Your Body:

Pay attention to how different foods make you feel. If certain foods enhance your energy levels and well-being, consider incorporating them into your regular diet. Conversely, if you notice discomfort or sluggishness, adjust accordingly.

Conclusion: Nourishing Your Body, Energizing Your Practice:

In conclusion, fueling your Wall Pilates journey is a multifaceted endeavor that involves nourishing your body with nutrient-dense foods, staying hydrated, and adopting mindful eating practices. By integrating these nutrition tips into your daily routine, you'll not only enhance your physical performance but also support your overall well-being. Remember, nutrition is a dynamic and individualized aspect of wellness, so listen to your body, make adjustments as needed, and enjoy the transformative power of combining optimal nutrition with the practice of Wall Pilates.